SAY GOOD-BYE TO ILLNESS

BY

DEVI S. NAMBUDRIPAD
D.C., L.Ac., R.N., Ph.D.

BEST SELLING AUTHOR OF
"FREEDOM FROM ALLERGY"

and

"YOU CAN REPROGRAM YOUR BRAIN
TO PERFECT HEALTH"

THIS BOOK WILL REVOLUTIONIZE THE
PRACTICE OF MEDICINE

*" The doctor of the future will give no medicine,
but will interest his patients in the care of the
human frame, in diet and in the cause and
prevention of disease"*

Attributed to Thomas Alva Edison

Published By

DELTA PUBLISHING COMPANY
7282 Melrose Street, Suite F
Buena Park, CA 90621
(714) 739-2219

DEDICATION

This book is dedicated to
my loving husband, Kris Nambudripad
and
my beloved son, Roy

Library of Congress Catalog Card Number: 93-72169
ISBN Number: 0-9637570-0-8
Printed in U.S.A.

ACKNOWLEDGMENTS

I am deeply grateful to my husband, Kris K. Nambudripad, for his inspiration, encouragement and assistance in my schooling, and later, in the formulation of this project. Without his cooperation in reference work, revision of manuscripts, word processing and proofreading, it is doubtful whether this book would ever have been completed. My sincere thanks also to the people who have entrusted their care to me, for without them I would have had no technique and, obviously, this book would not have been written.

I am also deeply grateful to Karen Watts, Mary Karaba, Meg Brazil, Helen Tanner, Shirley Reason, Jean Elston, Grace Weber, Joyce Baisden and Helene Singer for believing in me from the very beginning of this research until the present -- by supporting my theory and helping me to conduct the continuing detective work. I also have to express my thanks to my twelve-year-old son, Roy, who assisted me in many ways in writing this book. Roy was a very sick baby, through whom I perfected my technique in the beginning of my search for an allergy cure. He is a healthy twelve-year-old youngster now. Additionally, I wish to thank M. Sreedharan at Delta Printers and Saji Abraham who designed the cover page for their help in and finalizing this project and Carol Bergin for her efforts in editing and formatting.

As for further acknowledgments, I am deeply grateful for my professional training; that is, the knowledge and skills acquired in classes and seminars on chiropractic and applied kinesiology at the Los Angeles College of Chiropractic in Whittier, California; the California Acupuncture College, Westwood Boulevard, Los Angeles, California; SAMRA University of Oriental Medicine, Beverly Boulevard, Los Angeles, California; and the clinical experience obtained at the clinics attached to these colleges.

My special thanks also go to Dr. Richard F. Farquhar at Farquhar Chiropractic Clinic, Alondra Boulevard, Bellflower, California; where under Dr. R.F. Farquhar I had many hours of special instructions and hands-on practice on kinesiology. I also acknowledge my gratitude for a series of Total Body Modification seminars under Dr. Victor Frank; and the series of Activator methods seminars under Dr. Arlan Fuhr. They are responsible for my own health, as I have indicated before, and for the health of thousands of my patients.

Many of the doctors of Western medicine, Oriental medicine, chiropractic, osteopathy, as well as nutritionists instrumental in this process, were professors at the institutions I have mentioned. Their willingness to give of themselves to teach, as well as their willing commitment of personal time to the interviews necessary to complete this work, places them beyond mere expressions of gratitude. They are servants to the greatest ideals of the medical profession.

FOREWORD

"You need to see Dr. Devi," I was told while I was waiting to be seen by another doctor. "Why?" I asked in a frustrated tone of voice. By that time, I was pretty fed up with doctors even though I was one myself. I had suffered from chronic fatigue syndrome for the past year and a half. To top it off, I had been hospitalized with my first attack of asthma and had been placed on very high doses of steroids, antibiotics and four different bronchodilators (the very substances I was accustomed to helping my patients successfully discontinue). No one seemed to know the cause of my medical condition.

After "escaping" from the hospital, I contacted an acupuncturist who was able to get me off the medications. However, I was at a standstill, unable to work because of the asthma and chronic fatigue. The acupuncturist (not my internist nor pulmonary specialist) had given me a "peak flow meter" to monitor my progress. For over three months the meter seemed stuck on 300 (normal for me is 500). Within fifteen to thirty minutes after eating my allergic foods, the meter would fall to 250. This was my first clue in identifying many of the foods or environments that were adversely affecting me. Finally, I travelled to Los Angeles for help.

"Yes, you must see Dr. Devi. She takes away allergies." "Takes away allergies?" I said in disbelief. "That's impossible! I'm a clinical ecologist, and I've treated allergies for years. You can't take them away. You can make people better by giving them shots or drops under the tongue but you don't take the allergy away. You just make them less sensitive or reactive." I said in my "doctor-know-it-all-attitude." Fortunately, however, I was so sick and desperate that I followed the suggestion.

Dr. Nambudripad's waiting room was filled with people, all with incredible stories of the results of her "Allergy Elimination Treatment." Although skeptical, I began to have hope. As Dr. Devi began testing me, using clinical kinesiology, I was shocked to find that I was reacting to many vitamins and minerals including vitamin C, B complex, zinc, iron, vitamin A, table salt and other essential nutrients of my every day diet. Most foods were causing problems. One by one, she began eliminating them using her special treatment technique and, to my amazement, in just nine days my peak flow meter rose 140 points and remained there even upon returning to my Colorado home with an altitude of 6000 feet. Then vitamins and other nutrients, instead of causing problems, were able to be assimilated and begin repairing damaged cells. Foods which had been a problem before did not even budge the peak flow meter. More importantly, I was able to return to work within a few days and have continued to heal.

An allergic reaction is simply an improper response of the immune system to an otherwise harmless substance, such as foods, vitamins, medications, pollen, flowers, weeds, grasses, trees, dust, formaldehydes, plastics, metals, etc. The body reacts by releasing powerful chemicals that cause classic symptoms such as runny nose, watery eyes, rashes, depression, anger, asthma, fatigue, headaches, insomnia and various pains in almost any part of the body. She pointed out to me that many health problems in people all over the world are undiagnosed allergic reactions or due to the lowering of the immune system by multiple allergic reactions that allow diseases to attack the weakened host.

A few months later I was privileged to attend a seminar taught by Dr. Nambudripad and learn how to implement the Nambudripad's Allergy Elimination Techniques in my office. The practice of medicine hasn't been the same ever since. What a thrill to treat a patient for an allergy to a B complex and see her hip pain of 40 years' duration disappear instantly!

Obtaining a patient medical history takes on a different meaning as Dr. Nambudripad teaches the art of detective sleuthing. Rarely do I recommend a supplement or vitamin without first testing to check for allergy of effectiveness. Eliminating allergies to medications allows the medicines to be more effective while you are tracking down and eliminating the cause of the problems. Once the cause has been found, it may be no longer necessary to take the medication.

Certain patterns have been observed by practitioners of NAET (Nambudripad's Allergy Elimination Treatment) and provide useful protocols for helping our patients. For example, those suffering from arthritis should be checked for allergy to table salt, corn products, peppers, nutmeg, other spices and dried beans. The people who are troubled with clinical depression, without any help from known anti-depressants should be checked for the allergy to B complex vitamins, sugar, and trace minerals. Those plagued with addictions to alcohol, drugs, chocolate, caffeine or cigarettes are shown to be helped easier if allergy to vitamin B complex and sugars are eliminated prior to treating the allergy to the addicting substance.

Many symptoms and diseases are very often tied in one way or another to allergies to seemingly harmless substances in our environment. One person's chronic cough was relieved by eliminating an allergy to her lipstick. One woman had suffered hypertension for many years and yet was on a good diet, exercised daily and had a positive attitude. Extensive searching finally revealed the culprit: an allergy to nylon, she has remained normotensive for several months...goodbye hypertension. Since that case, I have discovered and successfully treated three people with hypertension related to allergy to nylon. A telephone operator's eczema disappeared when NAET was done on the plastics found in her keyboard.

Anyone who has tried to wrestle with an elimination or rotation diet knows how frustrating that can be, not only for yourself, but especially for school age children. How wonderful it is to know that one doesn't have to give up allergic items such as wheat, corn, chocolate, home and furnishings, the family pets, one's favorite clothes, the job that one loves, the perfumes, the make-up items or the computers that one depends upon for one's livelihood, etc., by doing such an easy, painless treatment!

Thank you Dr. Nambudripad for persevering in the development and documentation of this fantastic Allergy Elimination Technique. I also applaud you for the countless hours you spend in teaching the patients to test themselves and determine hidden allergies that might be causing trouble. Giving the patients that information helps them to take responsibility for their own health and puts them in charge instead of in the role of a victim. Then patient and doctor can work together as a team to achieve a mutual goal; of course, to "Say Good-bye To Illness" by reprogramming the brain to optimal health!

Sandra C. Denton, M.D.
Alaska Alternative Medicine Center
4115 Lake Otis Parkway, Suite 200
Anchorage, Alaska 99508

TABLE OF CONTENTS

PREFACE

I suffered since childhood from a multitude of health problems. It is no wonder then, that because of this prolonged and first-hand knowledge of ill health, I became focused on health-related problems, particularly those related to allergies. This undoubtedly resulted in following my natural inclination to pursue medicine as a profession. Eventually, I became a registered nurse, a chiropractor, a kinesiologist and an acupuncturist. I began specializing in treatment of the allergic patient, using methods I learned through intensive study of Oriental medicine, combined with the more traditional methods learned from my training as a nurse and its Western tradition.

It was during my studies and early practice as an allergist, when I began using eclectic methods of allergy treatments, that I arrived at the discovery that has ultimately resulted in my own good health. The integration of the relevant techniques from the various fields I studied, combined with my own discoveries, have since become the focus of my practice. There is no known successful method of treatment for food allergies, using Western medicine, except avoidance, which means deprivation and frustration.

The new technique of allergy elimination, which I have developed to treat food, as well as environmental allergies, was developed by combining the knowledge I received from three fields of Medicine. Kinesiology is the art and science of movement of the human body; comparing the movement of any muscle, one can measure the weakening effect of an allergy. Chiropractic medicine gives us the knowledge of the importance of maintaining the flow of nerve energy; a pinched nerve or an obstruction in the energy flow can cause a disease in the human body. Acupuncture teaches the importance of maintaining homeostasis in the body; any disturbance in the homeostasis can cause disease. Hence, diseases can be prevented and cured by maintaining an absolute balanced state of energy circulation in the body.

As an infant, I had severe infantile eczema, which lasted until I was seven or eight years old. Until then, I was fed Western medicine and Ayurvedic herbal medicine every day of my life, without a break. (Ayurveda is the traditional Indian system of medicine, based largely on herbs and naturopathy.) Western medicine did not help me at all; herbal medicine helped me somewhat. While I was taking the herbal medicines, my symptoms were under control; whenever I went off the herbs, my eczema recurred.

When I was eight years old, one of the herbal doctors told my parents to feed me white rice cooked with some special herbs. This special diet helped me a great deal. In a few months my eczema cleared up. But my good health did not last too long. I started to have symptoms of arthritis. On certain days, all my joints ached, and I stayed in bed for days at a time. Whenever I ate the white rice cooked with herbs I felt better. So, I started liking white rice more and more, because it made me feel better. Thus, white rice became the staple diet for me.

In 1976, when I came to Los Angeles, I became more health-conscious and tried to change my eating habits to eat more whole grain products and complex carbohydrates. All of a sudden I became very ill. I suffered from bronchitis and pneumonia and my arthritis returned. This became severe. I suffered from insomnia, clinical depression, constant sinusitis and frequent migraine headaches. I felt extremely tired all the time, but, when I went to bed, I remained wide awake. I tried many different medicines, changed doctors, antibiotics and consulted nutritionists. All the medicines, vitamins and herbs made me sicker, and the good nutrition made me worse. I was nauseated all the time. Every inch of my body ached. I lived on aspirin, taking almost 30 aspirin a day to keep me going.

During this time, I had three miscarriages, which broke me down emotionally. In order to keep my sanity, I decided to go back to school, coughing and puffing my way through. Following my mother's advice, I became very religious and began to observe all the religious holidays. I fasted, with only water intake, on all the Hindu religious holy days. The day after the fast I felt better, had more energy and my mind was clearer. As a result, I took more and more interest in fasting. I thought, "Fasting is a sacrifice; I am doing this in God's name and that is why I feel better the day after the fast." I know now that staying away from foods, to which I was allergic, during the fast was the reason for my feeling of well-being the next day.

During this time, I started my medical school training at the Los Angeles College of Chiropractic. By then, I had been fighting an attack of chronic bronchitis for two years. My nutrition teacher advised me to go on a juice diet. In two days, I had laryngitis, my bronchitis got worse and I had a fever of 104 degrees Fahrenheit. I stayed home for three days eating cooked soft white rice. In the southern part of India where I come from, cooked soft rice was the only food one ate when one got sick with a common cold or a fever. So I did the same and finally almost recovered from that episode.

When I returned to college, we had a guest speaker, who was an acupuncturist. I was sitting in a corner of the classroom coughing frequently. He watched me for a while and commented that I was suffering from an attack of wind/heat (common cold in Chinese medicine). I did not understand at the time what he meant by that phrase. He explained a few things about acupuncture and gave me a quick treatment using acupressure on acupuncture points. His treatments made me feel very good, and I quit coughing. I had heard about acupuncture before, but now I got first hand knowledge. I felt very happy to learn about this new branch of medicine and I was impressed with it, because it gave me some relief from my nagging symptoms.

All of a sudden my mind was thinking only of acupuncture. I went to the guest speaker, got the address of an acupuncture college, called the school the same day and signed up for classes.

The very first class was in acupressure. My teacher decided to teach muscle response testing to detect food allergies that day. By then my cough had returned. He noticed my chronic raspy cough, and he suspected that I was suffering from food allergies. He then tested me for various allergies to food items through muscle response testing. I reacted to almost everything he tested, except for white rice and broccoli. He suggested that I might do better if I only ate white rice and broccoli exclusively for a few days.

By then, I had been examined and treated by many doctors including, neurologists, cardiologists, psychologists, nutritionists and herbalists. Nobody suspected allergies as a cause of my chronic ill health. I was excited by this new knowledge. I was willing to try anything to get better. I followed my teacher's advice and ate white rice and broccoli exclusively. Within one week's time, my bronchitis cleared, my headaches became infrequent and less intense, my joints eased and my back did not hurt anymore. My thinking and concentration became clearer. My two year old depression disappeared. I did not have insomnia anymore. My general, body aches cleared. For the first time in my life, I experienced pain-free days. Until then, I was under the impression that everybody was supposed to have a certain amount of body aches and pains all the time, because I had never known otherwise. It was a treat for me to go to bed without pain and wake up in the morning with out pain.

After a week's restricted diet, I tried eating some other foods. My previous complaints slowly began to conquer me. I went on eating a white rice and broccoli diet. This time, I ate this food for three and a half years. Once in a while, I might try a bite of other foods, but my arthritic symptoms would return. I could not eat salads, fruits or vegetables, because I was very allergic to vitamin C. I could not eat whole grain products because they contained B complex. I could not eat fruits, honey, or any products made from sugars. These made me extremely tired, because I was very allergic to sugar. I could not drink or eat milk or milk products, because I was very allergic to calcium. I was highly allergic to fish groups, because I was allergic vitamin A. I was allergic to egg products, because eggs gave me skin problems. I was allergic to all types of beans, including soybeans, they gave me severe joint pains. Spices gave me arthritis of all the small joints. Almost all the fabrics, except silk, gave me itching, joint pain, and extreme tiredness. My teacher at the acupuncture college confirmed my doubts. I was just simply allergic to everything under the sun, including the sun by radiation.

A few years ago, in India, I complained to one of my doctors about my constant body aches and electric-shock like sensations in the body and in turn he diagnosed me as suffering from "hysteria" and having psychosomatic disorders. I felt very sad at that diagnosis, because I knew that I had no hysteria or psychosomatic disorders but real pain. I hoped and prayed that someday, somehow, I would get relief of my pain. Now I know all about "hysteria," it is simply a scapegoat diagnosis of frustrated doctors, who have not learned to diagnose their patients, or do not know how to find the causes of their patients' actual problems.

It seemed that I was allergic to everything except white rice, broccoli, silk and aspirins. What a combination! At least I was lucky to have a few items I was not allergic to. In my practice, I see many people with allergies to everything one could think of. Most of them were living in a place equivalent to a bubble before they were treated with Nambudripad's Allergy Elimination Treatments. When one is allergic to almost everything around (food, drinks, polluted air, chemicals, fabrics, living environments, etc.), it usually takes one to two years of continuous treatments, with Nambudripad's Allergy Elimination Treatments (two - three sessions a week), before they can come out of their bubble to the real world with pollution, fumes, chemicals, formaldehyde, pesticides, smog, etc.

I was very happy to live with few limited nonallergenic items. I lived eating white rice and broccoli for three and a half years. Then, one day around noon, when I came home from work, I ate a few pieces of carrots, while I was waiting for the rice to cook. In a few minutes, I felt tired and lethargic, and I soon felt like I was going to pass out. I tested myself with the carrots, using muscle response tests for allergies, and found I was highly allergic to them. I had already eaten three to four carrot sticks by then. My husband was working on his computer in the adjoining room. I called out to him for help and asked him to bring me the acupuncture needles from the study. I was very weak, light-headed and I didn't trust myself walking to the study to get the needles.

Meanwhile, I massaged the specific revival acupuncture points on my body, to prevent my fainting, and to keep myself awake until the needles arrived. I needled myself in all the important points that I knew would keep me from fainting, or from going into an anaphylactic shock. After inserting the needles, I slept for 45 minutes. When I woke up I felt strangely different. I was not sick or tired anymore. Instead, I felt a renewed pleasant energy. I didn't understand why. I had taken needles before for food reactions but had never felt like this. When I got up from the bed, I found that a few pieces of carrots were still stuck on me. I had a bunch of them in my hand, while I was getting the reaction. In a panic, I had dropped the carrots on the bed. I had been lying on them accidentally during the needle treatment.

Suddenly, I wondered whether there could be any connection between my feeling of supreme well-being, and carrots being in my electromagnetic field, while I was having the treatment. During those days I was taking a class in "electromagnetic field and acupuncture" at college. This helped me to understand the connection between the electromagnetic force of my body and the carrots. We were taught in the class that every object on the earth, whether living or non-living, has an energy field around it. It is attracted to the earth, because the earth has its own energy field. All these different energies can attract themselves or repulse from each other depending upon the difference of the energies.

I tested the carrots for allergy and was OK. I ate one whole carrot stick and did not have any reaction. I tried some other foods I was known to be allergic to, and reacted as before, so I knew my assumption was correct. My allergy to carrots was cured because of my contact with the sample while undergoing Acupuncture. My energy and the carrot's energy were repulsing before the acupuncture.

The repulsive energy between my body and the carrot appeared as an allergy. During the acupuncture treatment, my body probably became a powerful charger and was strong enough to change the adverse charge of the carrot to match with my charge. This resulted in removing my carrot allergy. I continued to treat for other items that I could not eat. I tested and treated my husband and my son. In a few weeks, we were no longer allergic to many foods that once made us ill. We could eat and enjoy a variety of foods without getting sick. Later, I extended this to my patients who suffered from a multitude of symptoms that arose from allergies.

My amazing recovery and return to health has now been duplicated over and over in my patients. I am convinced that I have discovered something truly wonderful about the treatment of allergies that does not include strict diets, stringent potions of any kind or isolation to avoid the allergy-producing environmental elements. It is this knowledge, as well as the urgent prompting of thousands of my patients who no longer suffer from symptoms of their allergies, that prompted the writing of this book.

The more extensively I studied the subject of allergies, the more I found it to be a truly fascinating, yet highly complex field. I also discovered that, although it has been gaining acceptance as a separate area of medical study in the last few years, it certainly has not been given the recognition it deserves as a primary cause of many types of disorders and illnesses. In fact, knowledge of the field is still quite limited among the general public. Even those whose primary practice is in the treatment of allergies, recognize the limitations due to the comparatively small amount of research that has been done in the field.

After learning about the prevalence of allergies, and gathering a great deal of clinical, hands-on experience with patients, I felt motivated to write a book on allergies that might be of use to students and professionals in the health care field. However, as I thought about the book, I came to understand that good health care really depends on the patient. Therefore, it is just as imperative to inform the general public about allergies as it is to educate the health-care professional. So, this book is written not only for the health-care professional but also for lay persons wishing to acquire an understanding of the allergic process taking place within the body.

The framework, or skeleton, on which the book is developed is drawn from a formal dissertation I submitted to SAMRA University of Oriental Medicine, Los Angeles, in June of 1986, as a basis for my doctorate degree. It differs from the doctoral dissertation not only in length, structure, and style but also with respect to contents and focus. The principal difference is the fact that a dissertation is typically a scholarly treatise. Accordingly, my dissertation was a comparison of the oriental with the modern Western medical approach to the treatment of patients suffering from allergic reactions. Technical terminology was used throughout.

This book, on the other hand, has been condensed and popularized and is written with a different thrust. That is, it is designed first to provide up-to-date information about the current state-of-the art in allergic treatment; second, to create a book that can be of value to people suffering from allergic symptoms; and third, to enhance the reader's knowledge and understanding of allergic reactions and possible alternative treatment methods.

I am aware that technical terminology or jargon is a part of any highly specialized field. After all, technical terminology is necessary for the professional, because it reduces the need for unnecessary, explanatory words and clarifies instructions. It is also clear that use of technical jargon severely reduces the ability of the uninitiated to understand important facts. Thus, the technical jargon developed around any highly technical field actually creates a significant communication barrier between the professional and the lay person.

In this book, since the specialized terminology may give some lay readers a difficult time and severely diminish their reading pleasure (let alone, their understanding), technical terms are kept to a minimum, with apologies to the professional reader.

Caution has also been exercised in deciding on the depth to which various aspects of the subject matter should be taken. For instance, an understanding is only just now being arrived at as to how allergies and nervous system are inextricably interrelated. But since the human nervous system is one of the most complex areas of the human anatomy and remains largely uncharted, it was decided to deal with it in a sweeping fashion, drawing the readers' attention only to the close link between the nervous system and allergic reactions.

I would feel gratified indeed if the up-to-date material compiled in this book were to contribute to the reader's achieving, maintaining and enjoying good health; and if through these readers, an even larger number of people were meant to receive benefits through methods that are available today.

To enhance your understanding of the subject matter, the reader is referred to the relevant books and articles, some of which are quoted as a part of this book. They are listed under the section on "BIBLIOGRAPHY" at the conclusion of this book.

Since the main stay of this presentation is acupuncture and, since not even a single aspect of a medical system should be practiced or talked about without some understanding of that medical system, it seems to me that an introduction to the basis of traditional Chinese medicine (TCM) is mandatory. It should be kept in mind, however, that an in-depth introduction to oriental medicine was neither intended nor considered appropriate within the scope of this publication. The reader is therefore urged to refer to appropriate books for more information. Some of the references are listed in the bibliography.

Los Angeles, California
Dr. Devi S. Nambudripad, D.C., L.Ac., R.N., Ph.D (Acu)
June, 1993

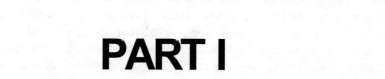

PART I

CHAPTER ONE

WHAT IS ALLERGY?

Over a period of ten years, Carolyn had been hospitalized a total of twelve times for seizure episodes, bronchitis, acute asthmatic attacks and frequent bouts of pneumonia. Each time she was hospitalized between a few days to a few weeks to recover from the acute problems. Gradually, over a period of a few weeks to several months, she recovered from the weakness. By the time she gained some strength, another episode of asthma or pneumonia placed her back in the hospital. She had been on disability for some ten years. A talented musician, she could not work or play music, even as a leisure activity.

She had tried everything she could think of to get help. Several physicians in general medicine had already given up trying to help her. She had been seen by an internist, a neurologist, a vascular surgeon, a lung specialist and by at least four doctors specializing in the treatment of allergies. She had undergone nearly every diagnostic procedure known to modern medicine. On the advice of one physician, she underwent psychiatric evaluation. Still, the ongoing headaches, asthmatic symptoms, muscle and joint pains, epileptic type seizures, persistent dry cough, post-nasal drip, chronic diarrhea, frequent bladder infections, yeast infections, frequent urination, dyslexia, frequent disorientation and extreme fatigue of body and mind persisted.

This is the story of a real person; who, like so many others around us, suffers the frustrating and agonizing symptoms of allergies. Symptoms that not only confuse and frustrate the patients and treating doctors but also place tremendous stress on the patients' families and employers.

The facts of this actual case history are not atypical. The hospitalization and heavy doses of Cortisone and antibiotics

Carolyn received help produce relief from the symptoms of allergies in a majority of allergic patients. However, the possibility of repeated episodes always waits around the corner. The side effects of Cortisone and other anti-allergenic medicines increase the risk of heart disease, obesity, joint disorders and moon face (a temporary deformity caused by allergic reactions to the drugs prescribed to reduce the original allergic syndromes, making the overall condition worse).

There is hardly a human disease or condition that may not involve an allergic factor. Further allergic studies and investigations are constantly revealing new conditions that are caused by various allergic reactions. Any organ, or group of organs, or any portion of the body may be involved, though the allergic responses may vary greatly.

The term "allergy" was first proposed in 1906 by an Austrian pediatrician, Clemens Von Pirquet (1874-1929), who worked a great deal with tubercular children and studied the immune system and what we now call allergic reactions. It was Pirquet who developed a scratch test for tuberculosis, a forerunner of the allergy scratch-testing done in many allergy clinics today. By combining the two Greek words *allos* (altered) and *ergion* (action or reactivity), Pirquet created the word "allergy," literally "altered reactivity," that is, a biological hypersensitivity in certain individuals to substances which, in similar amounts and circumstances, are innocuous for most other persons.

Although the term "allergy" has been used by the medical profession and the public for many decades, knowledge about the nature of allergies and their wide range and implications is still in an embryonic stage. Even in this enlightened age, many people, including some health professionals, on hearing the word "allergy" think only of a runny nose, sneezing, hives and perhaps asthma or hay fever. Fortunately, on the other hand, an increasing number of medical doctors and researchers now consider allergic factors may be involved in most illnesses and medical disorders.

Somewhere around mid-400 B.C., nearly 2500 years ago, Hippocrates, the Greek physician whom we call the "Father of Medicine," noted that cheese caused severe reactions in some men, while others could eat and enjoy it with no unpleasant after effects. Three hundred years later, the Roman philosopher, Lucretius said, "What is food for some may be fierce poison for others." From this observation has come our expression, "One man's meat is another man's poison." This is a simple and concise definition of allergy, although the condition was not recognized as such until very recently.

An allergy is a hereditary condition: an allergic predisposition or tendency is inherited but may not be manifested until some later date. Researchers have found that when both parents were or are allergy-sensitive, 75 to 100 percent of their offspring react to those same allergies. When neither of the parents is or was sensitive to allergens, a probability of producing allergic offspring drops dramatically to less than 10 percent.

It was also learned that in some cases, even when parents had no allergies, their offspring still suffered from many allergies since birth. In these cases, various possibilities exist: parents may have suffered from a serious disease or condition before the child was born that caused alteration in the genetic codes; the pregnant mother may have been exposed to harmful things like radiation, chemicals, drugs, or toxins as the result of a disease (strep throat, measles, chicken pox, etc.); or parents may have suffered severe malnutrition, possibly causing the growing embryo to undergo cell mutation during its development in the womb. The altered cells then do not carry over the original genetic codes or do not go through normal development. The organs and tissues which are supposed to develop from the effected cells remain non-functional.

4

Sometimes, due to this alteration, sensory nerve receptors or the nerve energy supply to certain organs remains dormant and is unable to conduct messages to and from the spinal cord and the brain. In some instances, these dormant receptors become hyposensitive toward certain items, whereas, in other people they become hypersensitive. Neither type functions normally.

In the group of people where dormant fibers turn hypersensitive, we often see enormous allergic reactions. In people where hyposensitive fibers are predominant, few allergic reactions may be seen, but we can see poor growth and poor functions of body and mind. We call the hypersensitivity "active allergies," and the hyposensitivity "hidden allergies." Both of these types can be tested positive by muscle response test (MRT), the test originally discovered by Dr. George Goodheart. Most other standard tests available today in the modern world to test allergies are unable to detect hidden allergies successfully. "Nambudripad's Allergy Elimination Techniques," started by Dr. Devi S. Nambudripad in 1983, can be used successfully to wake up the dormant sensory nerve fibers and thus restore normal functions of the body parts or organs, which those sensory nerve fibers supply. (Muscle-Response Tests and "Nambudripad's Allergy Elimination Techniques" will be described later.)

It has also been studied and proven that the age of onset of an allergic condition definitely depends on the degree of inheritance. Thus, the stronger the genetic factor, the earlier the probable onset.

In some people, the altered changes of the sensory nerve fibers may occur during their own lifetimes and may not be inherited. Major illnesses, severe reactions to drugs, toxins, chemicals, radiation, etc., are capable of causing damage to the sensory nerve fibers and marring their conductivity.

Such is the unique case of a 38-year-old female who manifested tremendous allergic reactions to a great many foods and objects in the environment. Her history revealed that when she was one-year-old, after a routine smallpox vaccination, she suffered a severe reaction and almost died. She did not show other allergic inheritance characteristics from her parents or grandparents, since all of them were very healthy. She suffered physical allergies such as hives, joint pains and migraines; gastrointestinal allergies such as indigestion, heart burn, intermittent chronic diarrhea or constipation; emotional reactions such as depression, anger, crying spells, lacking interest in day-to-day activities, severe pre-menstrual syndromes, etc., for many years. When she was treated for small pox vaccination by Nambudripad's Allergy Elimination Techniques, she was able to clear her allergic reactions to various items. Her physical, physiological and emotional symptoms changed toward normal very quickly after the treatment.

There is no limit to the number and kinds of substances that cause allergic reactions. Any substance under the sun, including sunlight, can cause an allergic reaction in any individual. In our highly technological age, the number of substances that are potentially allergenic are constantly being expanded as we learn what it truly means to "live better through chemistry."

A substance capable of producing an allergic reaction is known as an allergen and, as mentioned previously, may be different for every person. For instance, most people, but not all, are allergic to poison oak or poison ivy. For the same reason, most people find roses to be nothing more than a beautiful and fragrant flower. No matter what the substance may be, it is an allergen for that single person in whom that substance produces an allergic reaction. In other words, it is the reaction to the substance that earns the recognition of allergen.

A 72-year-old female had chronic weeping ulcers on the tips of the fingers of both her hands for many years and had tried all the possible medicines and ointments on the stubborn ulcers. While taking her history, it was revealed that caring for roses was her main hobby. Having taken this into consideration, she was tested for the roses by muscle response testing and was found to be highly allergic to them. When she was treated by Nambudripad's Allergy Elimination Techniques for allergies, her chronic ulcers healed nicely.

Although the word "allergy" has been described above, further explanation is necessary to understand the changes that actually take place in the body when an allergic manifestation occurs. An allergy is an unusual or exaggerated response to certain substances. It is believed to be a normal response that has been abnormally exaggerated.

For instance, when an inflammation of the eye occurs, it is probably an effort on the part of the eye to throw off some irritating substance. When the nose begins to drip and the hay fever victim sneezes, this is an effort on the part of these organs to eliminate some of the irritants (such as pollen) causing the irritation. When giant hives occur, watery fluid becomes present in the tissues, probably for the purpose of washing away what-ever substance is causing the trouble. When asthma occurs, the bronchial tubes contract in an effort to prevent the irritant from penetrating deeper into the lungs.

These reactions are controlled by the autonomous (automatic) nervous system, which is composed of the sympathetic and para-sympathetic nerves. They control such functions as the lachrymal glands, which secrete tears; the glands in the mouth, which secrete saliva; the respiratory organs, the digestive system and the heart. These automatic processes are controlled by the two systems of nerves which act antagonistically against each other. The sympathetic nerves cause relaxation in the muscles, and the parasympathetic nerves cause muscles to contract. When the two systems are functioning properly, we are not aware of these processes. When one system over balances the other, certain things occur in the body which make us aware of their existence.

For instance, when a person is frightened or angry, the adrenal glands secrete additional adrenalin into the bloodstream, which stimulates the activity of certain organs and tissues of the body. The heart works more rapidly, perspiration flows more freely, and the body summons all its defense forces to get protection and save the body from any possible damage (preparing the body for "fight or flight"). This happens when sympathetic nerves are in control, and under these conditions no allergic symptoms occur.

According to Oriental medical principals, this is the state of "free flowing of energy" of the energy pathways. Free flowing of energy ensures the perfect balance of the body. When the body is in perfect balance, no allergic reaction or disease is possible. In fact, persons who have severe allergic symptoms, such as asthma, do not have these symptoms when they are very angry or very frightened. It is a well known fact that on a battle-field even chronic asthmatics have no symptoms whatsoever. It is this knowledge of what adrenalin accomplishes for people suffering from allergic symptoms that has formed the basis of our modern knowledge and use of adrenalin as a drug in treating allergic patients.

The parasympathetic nerves, which act in the opposite manner, contract rather than relax the muscles. They can also cause relaxation of vigilance on the part of certain organs, such as the blood vessels, which become more permeable when these nerves are in control. When asthma occurs, the bronchial tubes are contracted and the air is prevented from escaping, as it should and does, in normal breathing. When giant hives occur, it is because proper control of the blood vessels have been relaxed and become more permeable, permitting fluid to escape into the tissues.

Illness is a warning given by the brain to the rest of the body of the organism regarding energy blockages within the energy channels of the organism. Through illness, pain, inflammation, fever, heart attacks, strokes, abnormal growths, tumors and various discomforts, the brain signals the body about the possible dangers if the energy blockages are allowed to continue within the channels. If the symptoms are minor, blockages are minor. If the symptoms are major, the blockages are major. Minor blockages can be unblocked easily, whereas major blockages take a long time to unblock.

Through 31 pairs of spinal nerves, the brain operates the largest network of communication within the body. Energy blockages happen in a person's body due to contact with adverse energy of other substances. When two adverse energies come closer, repulsion takes place. When two similar energies get together, attraction takes place. The repulsion of energies is referred to in this book as allergy.

The repulsion of energies can happen between two living organisms, (e.g., between two humans, such as father and son; two siblings, husband and wife; two friends, animal and human being etc.,). It can also occur between one living organism and one non-living organism. For example, between a human being and fabrics or food; between one living organism and energies of other substances (i.e., food, a cat, other human beings like husband, mother, child, co-workers etc., fabrics, furniture, fumes, trees, pollens, chemicals, work materials, radiation from the television, microwave, radio, sun, etc.) at the same time.

When a person's energy tries to block other adverse energies at the same time, the person's energy becomes weaker against all other energies. The failure to overcome the attack of adverse energies causes the energy pathways of the weak body to create blocks toward all the adverse energies around it. The result, whenever an adverse energy comes close to the proximity, the energy pathways contract and become blocked. When such a person is surrounded by numerous adverse energies all the time, his/her energy pathways remain blocked all the time. The continuous blockage of the energy pathways causes poor body function. The blockages caused in a person's body from many sources at the same time can be larger and deeper. The symptoms resulting from such blockage can also be severe in intensity.

Lets try to understand the blocking process further. Robert, a 32-year-old computer programmer, had suffered from chronic fatigue syndrome for seven years and had been completely disabled for two years. He also had frequent headaches, joint pains, indigestion, pain in the abdomen and insomnia. He began working with computers ten years prior, married eight years ago and had two children, aged seven and five. He was found to be allergic to many things: eggs, milk, fruits, sugar, wheat, carrots, salt, corn, dried beans, spices, polyester, synthetic fabrics, chemical fumes, trees, grasses, his dog, inks, ceramics, computer, plastics, keyboards, computer radiation, formaldehyde, his wife and one child.

Lets evaluate each allergen separately and how they individually contributed toward his disability. Food products are taken by mouth. When the food enters the digestive tract, the essence of food gets absorbed into various meridians and organs in the body and is used for various functions.

Eggs and dried beans: His body could not tolerate animal or vegetable proteins, from the time he was born, which made him less resistant toward various proteins. This in turn caused him to have a weak immune system. The human body depends on protein utilization and assimilation for normal everyday body functions, like protein synthesis, kreb cycle, fighting against foreign proteins like bacteria, viruses, etc.

Milk: Milk and milk products provide many essential nutrients, mainly calcium. Calcium is another essential item to keep our body healthy. Allergy to milk and milk products causes poor absorption of calcium.

Fruits and vegetables: Vitamin C is necessary to repair wear and tear of the body, to help keep a normal immune system and for normal growth and development.

Grains: Allergy to grains also caused him to be allergic to B complex vitamins. B vitamins are necessary for the normal functions of the nervous system. In the absence of B vitamins various enzymatic functions will not take place in the body.

Sugar: Sugar is another substance one needs in the body for normal functions. Energy is necessary for bodily functions. Sugar provides energy. If the body can not absorb or utilize sugar, most of the body functions suffer.

Iron: A person gets his iron from foods like raisins, nuts and meats, etc. When one is allergic to these food groups, iron absorption is impaired. Lack of iron makes the person anemic, among other things, and makes one tired.

Salt: Allergy to salt means allergy to one's body, because each and every cell of the body contains sodium. Integrity of the sodium - potassium pump depends on the ability of the absorption and utilization of the salts. The sodium-potassium pump keeps the body electrical. This electricity keeps the body alive.

Spices: Allergy to spices causes water retention and tissue swelling. Thus, this could cause headaches if the brain tissue gets affected by water retention and tissue swellings. If other joints get affected, then pain and swelling of the joints happen.

Chemicals: If one is allergic to chemicals, the adverse energy could penetrate into the body through skin, thus blocking the energy pathways. Adverse energy from chemicals could travel faster than anything else. This could produce tiredness, light-headedness, brain fog, sharp pains in the body etc., within a few seconds of exposure to the allergens. The same applies to fumes, formaldehydes, radiation, fabrics, etc.

Allergy to human beings and animals also works like a chemical allergy. When one is near the energy of allergic human beings or animals, the body tries to protect the person by creating blockages.

In the case of Robert, he was surrounded by the adverse energies of various foods from the time he was born. When he began working with the computers for hours and hours, the allergy to the computer material, along with radiation, added to the blockage. Then, the adverse energy of his wife came along and caused more blockages. His child added more to his agony. His body was constantly fighting various energy blockages, whether he was at work or home and whether he was aware of the blockages or not.

During this constant fight for survival, his body lost the battle and became physically ill and later disabled. When he finally retired in the house, his wife and other allergens were around him all the time. His condition got worse as the days progressed. Since there were many equally strong allergens around him, it was difficult to say which one affected him the most. He always felt sick. The reason for his illness was blamed on chronic fatigue syndrome or some virus attack....

When his allergies were removed one by one by Nambudripad's Allergy Elimination Technique, his blockages became fewer and fewer. He started feeling better most of the time. When most allergens were eliminated, his body began identifying other allergens. Those allergens have not been treated but bothered him nevertheless.

At this point, some people might wonder if he was getting more allergic to other things or if he was getting more sensitive to existing allergens. He was not getting more allergic to other things nor was he getting too sensitive to existing allergens.

First of all, he learned to look at his chronic illness in a different way. Until now, he was made to believe that there was no known cure for his debilitating disease, so he took it as his destiny to be sick. Now he was taught to look at all his health problems as the result of some allergies. His awareness got sharper. When he was living in the midst of allergens, he always felt sick and miserable. When he got himself freed of a few allergens and experienced a few good days and then experienced an allergen attack, he felt the affect stronger than before.

When the energy channels are filled with unblocked energy, and the energy circulates through the channels freely, the body is said to be in a perfect balance. In other words, we can say that the body is in homeostasis. When the body is in homeostasis, it can function normally and allergies do not affect the body. In this state, the body can absorb all the necessary nutrients from the food eaten.

The energy channels need energy to function normally. This energy is produced from the nutrients consumed, such as vitamins, minerals, sugars, etc. The attraction or repulsion of the electromagnetic energy field is created in the body by the interaction of the various charged nutrients inside the body. Each cell is an electricity generating unit. Each cell is loaded with positively charged potassium and some sodium. Most of the sodium is outside the cell. The sodium and potassium keep circulating in and out of the cell in the presence of water with the help of other nutrients like proteins and sugars. These charged molecules inside the body make the whole body an electrical unit with an electrical field around it.

Allergy, as stated in this chapter, is an unusual characteristic that causes energy blockages against other organisms or substances. In other words, this is an unusual sensitivity of one organism toward certain substances. This tendency to react physically in an unusual manner to various things is inherited.

Whenever a body becomes imbalanced, allergic manifestations appear. An imbalance may be caused by any one of a number of things. It may follow a serious accident, a major operation, a childhood disease (i.e., whooping cough, chickenpox, etc.), or an emotional shock (i.e., loss of loved ones or loss of a job or property, childhood molestation, betrayal, battering, cult victims, child abuse, etc.), or it may be that the patient has been exposed repeatedly to the particular hypersensitive allergens over a short period and the body's defenses have become exhausted due to overwork.

These symptoms may be more acute at certain times of the year, particularly when the allergy is caused by pollens, which are more prevalent during specific seasons. The symptoms may also be worse in certain locations and under certain conditions.

In looking at sensitivities to particular substances, it is rare for such allergy to be inherited. Rather, it is the TENDENCY to respond or react in an unusual manner to various things that is inherited. The tendency itself often recurs from one generation to another.

With this understanding, we can look at most hospitalized patients with acute health problems and their relationship to the food they consumed before getting sick. Statistics of heart attack victims show that many heart attacks take place after or during elaborate meals such as Thanksgiving, Christmas, New Year's Day, weddings, etc. Until recently, blame for these incidents was placed on emotional triggers. Few individuals tried to connect heart attacks with food allergies.

On emotional and sentimental occasions such as those mentioned above, an allergic person tries to eat one more bite of all the tasty foods. With the first bite of most allergic foods, the brain begins to block the energy channels to prevent the entrance of adverse energy of the food into the body. To accomplish this, the brain calls upon its defensive forces for protection. With the second bite, the rest of the defensive forces go to work to protect the body. The body finally runs out of its defense forces.

The sympathetic and parasympathetic nerves do not coordinate well and the highly blocked area or the weakest parts of the body give up first. If that happens to be the heart, the victim's heart instantly stops functioning or functions abnormally. If the lungs are the highly blocked area of the body, the patient can have an asthmatic attack. If the stomach is the weakest, the person may get an acute abdominal pain, or a related migraine headache. Chronic effects of stomach blockages can also affect the brain function. A person can demonstrate manic disorders, schizophrenic disorders, depressive disorders etc.

If the spleen is weak, the person can suffer from general body ache, nausea, extreme fatigue, etc. If the pancreas is affected, one can suffer from sugar intolerance or absorption problems like hypoglycemia, or diabetes. If the liver is weak, one can experience emotional imbalances, anger, mood swings, depression and premenstrual symptoms. If the kidneys are affected, one can become very fearful all the time and can suffer from various arthritis and chronic backaches. If the bladder is affected, one can suffer from yeast type infections, frequent urination and eye infections. If the colon is affected, one can suffer from latent asthma, knee pains, constipation and lower backache.

Lets follow the heart attack victim further. When he or she has a heart attack, someone calls the paramedics. If a lot of allergens have not been consumed, the victim may stay alive until help arrives. If he is not sensitive to the emergency drugs the paramedics inject, the heart attack victim will continue to breathe and function. In the cardiac unit he will be given complete rest from physical activities by being kept in bed, from emotional activities by sedation and from the ingestion of food allergens by abstinence from mouth feeding. In 48 to 72 hours, the allergic food will have a chance to get out of the body, the heart will begin to beat normally once again, and he or she will be labeled as out of danger.

On the other hand, if he or she was allergic to all or part of the drugs he received, his pains or symptoms may very well become progressively worse and the heart will eventually stop functioning. In these cases the last report will say: "In spite of all revival attempts, the patient expired."

Statistics also show that most sports injuries take place after food breaks or lunch periods. It is better to consume simple foods during sports sessions to avoid injuries.

CHAPTER TWO

CATEGORIES OF ALLERGENS

Allergens are generally classified into eight basic categories, depending primarily on the method in which they are contacted, rather than the symptoms they produce. They are: inhalants, ingestants, contactants, infectants, physical agents, genetic agents, molds, and fungi.

INHALANTS

Inhalants are those allergens that are contacted through the nose, throat and bronchial tubes. Examples of inhalants are microscopic spores of certain grasses, flowers, pollens, powders, smoke, cosmetics, perfumes; and chemical fumes such as paint, insecticides, fertilizers, flour from grains, etc.

It is difficult to say that there is a typical or predictable allergic reaction, or set of reactions, in response to a given allergen. If there is a predictable response, however, it is in this general category of inhalants that it comes closest to being found.

Most of us have suffered the discomfort that comes from accidentally breathing a toxic substance. For example, when we smell chlorine gas from a bottle of common household bleach, our reaction is immediate and violent as our eyes water, our noses run, and our bronchial tubes go into spasm, making breathing difficult. This experiment can be duplicated over and over if we want proof that bleach is directly responsible for a given set of reactions. Of course, most of us learn very quickly that it is the bleach that caused our discomfort, and we decide to be more careful in the future.

In this case, the cause of the discomfort (the bleach) was very closely associated with the effect, the burning eyes, runny nose, and restricted breathing. A simple and very scientific deduction, though slightly sophomoric in this context, can be drawn from this cause-and-effect relationship. A proper diagnosis based on a similar cause-and-effect relationship is much more difficult when the cause is olive pollen, encountered early in the day by one of the sensitive patients, and the resultant delayed effect is similar to that experienced when one breathes in the bleach. Similarly, hay fever is generally the result of breathing the spores of pollinating grass and weeds. It normally occurs when these plants are in bloom in the spring or, in warmer climates, closely following a summer rain and the resultant regrowth of the grasses and weeds on the hillsides. Sinus drainage and restricted breathing are the direct and reproducible results of an allergic reaction to an inhalant.

Consider how much more difficult it is to make a proper diagnosis when the patient's physical responses to a given allergen differ radically from those that would normally be anticipated. For instance, the case of a man in his early 60's who came to the author's office, nearly incapacitated by lapses of memory and seizures that resembled some form of epilepsy, Alzheimer's disease or perhaps a mild stroke. He would often wander off in total confusion or complete amnesia, sometimes losing track of significant blocks of time.

Neurological examination and a CAT scan showed his brain-wave pattern to be completely normal. After considerable detective work, the cause in this case turned out to be the airborne spores of a fern tree he had recently planted in his backyard. His reaction to the inhalant was totally illogical physiologically and unanticipated. The lack of respiratory distress seen in other patients, who suffer sensitivities to inhalants, delayed diagnosis and treatment for several months. This added to the frustration and potential danger to the patient.

This clearly points out that there is no typical response to allergens in the real world. If we are depending on allergies to produce a given set of responses for all people, we may mis-diagnose and provide wrong treatments. We must remember that since we cannot duplicate and package a cause-and-effect respon-sive medication as antidote to handle all cases of poisoning from inhaling fern tree spores or any other allergen, we must not over-simplify our treatment of patients who do not exhibit typical allergic symptoms, whatever we perceive them to be. In doing so, we risk missing myriad potential reactions that may be pro-duced in some people in response to their contacts with sub-stances that are, for them, allergens.

INGESTANTS

Ingestants are allergens that are contacted in the normal course of eating a meal or that enter the system in other ways through the mouth and, thus, find their way into the gastrointestinal tract. These include foods, condiments, drugs, beverages, chewing gums, vitamin supplements, etc. We must not ignore the poten-tial reactions to things that may be touched and inadvertently transmitted into the mouth by our hands.

It is also believed that many of the symptoms we know as alcoholism are the result of an allergy to alcohol, B-complex vitamins and sugars. Human brain function depends on sugar absorption and utilization. Sugar digestion and assimilation depends on certain enzymes made from B-complex in the body. When one has an allergy to B-complex and sugar, he or she may have the tendency to become addicted to alcohol. Alcohol can absorb into the tissue by osmosis. Alcohol consumption thus satisfies the brain's partial need for sugar -- temporarily.

Therefore, alcoholics indulge in drinking more and more to satisfy the need for sugar, a need that eventually turns into a dependency. This applies to 50 percent of alcoholics. The other 50 percent may fall into the group of people who become alcoholics due to certain pressures, such as peer pressure, boredom, social obligations, etc. These individuals turn out to be habitual drinkers -- but not alcoholics. If they ever make up their minds, it is easy for them to quit drinking without withdrawal symptoms.

People who are allergic to alcohol have severe withdrawal symptoms when they try to quit drinking. Sometimes, suppression of the desire to drink may turn into physical or psychological problems. Such was the case of a woman who tried to quit drinking by joining Alcoholics Anonymous. She ended up having severe neck pains, migraines and brachial neuralgia. A year and 18 months after she quit drinking, but she still suffered severe back pain. After she was treated by Nambudripad's Allergy Elimination Technique for sugar, B-complex, and alcohol allergies, she obtained relief of her chronic upper backache and migraines.

Another patient, a 52-year-old male, quit drinking 15 years ago when he joined AA. However, ever since he quit drinking, he had a chronic constant lower backache. He tried different treatments, including massage therapy, physical therapy, acupuncture, etc., with no relief. When he was treated by Nambudripad's Allergy Elimination Technique for alcohol, his 15-year-old backache improved.

The area of ingested allergens is one of the most difficult to diagnose, because the allergic responses are often delayed from several minutes to several days, making the direct association between cause and effect very difficult. This is not to say that an immediate response is not possible. Some people can react violently in seconds after they consume the allergens. In extreme cases, one has to only touch or come near the allergen to signal the central nervous system that it is about to be poisoned, result-ing in symptoms that are peculiar to that particular patient.

Usually more violent reactions are observed in ingested allergens than in other forms.

Such was the case of a young man in his early teens, who had come to the author's office for a sports-related injury. He also had a history of asthma. On one occasion his mother brought to the doctor's attention the fact that her son had some continuous itching in an area four finger widths below the knee, on the outer side of the anterior tibial crest. The itching was on the stomach meridian, which meant that the cause of the allergic rash was related to something he was eating. On questioning him further, it was revealed that whenever he ate his favorite breakfast cereal he broke out in a rash.

A simple experiment was set up to test and confirm it. He was given all his breakfast items: juice, toast and rice cereal, one by one. Then he was given time to chew. It all went well until he placed one, and only one, rice cereal flake in his mouth. He immediately complained of feeling hot and began to redden in an allergic rash, and in a few more seconds he had almost slipped into an anaphylactic shock. After several tense minutes and continuous treatment by Nambudripad's Allergy Elimination Technique, his symptoms subsided.

In a similar, but unfortunately more tragic instance, peanuts were responsible for the death of an otherwise healthy 12-year-old boy in the midwestern United States. Although he knew that he was allergic to peanuts, he accidentally ate them as an ingredient in cookies after a little league game. He died shortly after reaching the hospital in anaphylactic shock.

Literally any substance we eat can and does become an allergen for someone. For instance, people have been known to faint every time they eat an orange without exhibiting any other food allergies. By avoiding this allergen they can prevent the occurrence of an allergic reaction and may find it unnecessary to subject themselves to regular medical care. However, one should keep in mind that in this and in similar minor allergy cases, patients who are not treated tend to manifest allergic symptoms to other similar allergens. For instance, a patient who fainted when she ate an orange might develop asthma or migraine headaches when she eats a banana at a later date.

One of the patients in the author's clinic identified oranges as the one and only allergen that affected her. She complained that she was developing additional allergies to foods such as bananas, grape juice and squash. During routine testing for allergies, it was discovered that a single element in oranges, in fairly high concentration, was potassium. Because she had let the orange allergy go untreated, the potassium was untreated. Because the potassium was untreated, she began to react to other foods that contained potassium, even though it was a lower concentration in these foods.

She is really fortunate that she did not run into a recipe that called for a large amount of cream of tartar. This food additive is potassium bitartrate, and has many uses, including that of stiffener in meringue for pies and candies, presenting another problem for allergic patients.

We live in a highly technological age. New substances are being introduced into our diets that preserve color, flavor and extend the shelf life of our foods. There are some additives used in foods as preservatives that have caused severe health problems. Some artificial sweeteners cause mysterious problems in some people and may mimic various serious diseases such as multiple sclerosis, acute prostatitis, trigeminal neuralgia, vertigo, chronic dry cough, joint pains and sciatica, to name a few. Most of these additives are harmless to most people but can be fatal to some who react to these substances.

One 49-year-old man had seven years of longstanding urinary problems. He had frequent urination, especially at night, so that he had to get up at least 10 to 12 times a night, which gave him no rest. An elementary school teacher, he felt very tired most of the time due to lack of sleep. He was seen by urologists many times, and he had tried various antibiotics for a possible urinary tract infection and prostatitis. None of the medicines worked for him and his problem persisted. He was desperate and gave up teaching for a while.

When he came to our office, he was absolutely miserable. His history revealed that in the morning he had drank two to three cups of coffee with an artificial sweetener. He always had a couple of tuna sandwiches at night between 8 and 10 p.m. Further testing confirmed that he was highly allergic to artificial sweeteners and the sweet relish in the tuna sandwiches contained artificial sweeteners, which caused him to have frequent urination throughout the night. After he was treated by Nambudripad's Allergy Elimination Technique for artificial sweeteners, his long standing problem was solved.

A 24-year-old female complained that her hands fell asleep when ever she slept. She suffered from this unique problem for the past nine weeks. With the kinesiological diagnostic technique it was discovered that she was eating cream filled arrowroot cookies every night before she went to bed. When she was treated for the cookies, her hands did not fall asleep when she went to bed.

A 24-year-old woman was diagnosed as having multiple sclerosis. She had the typical symptoms of multiple sclerosis, numb hands, frequent headaches, bilateral lack of strength in the arms, extreme fatigue, shaking, weakness of the lower limbs, etc. She was on a diet to lose weight for six months, which was when her present symptoms started. During this time, she consumed lots of artificial sweeteners to which she was found to be highly allergic. When she was treated by Nambudripad's Allergy Elimination Technique for artificial sweeteners, these symptoms disappeared.

Another 67-year-old woman went to dinner at her diabetic brother's house. His wife had made rice pudding with artificial sweeteners. At about 10 p.m. she started to have excruciating pain on the right side of her face, which did not respond to any usual pain medications. She was treated for artificial sweeteners by Nambudripad's Allergy Elimination Technique, and her facial neuralgia diminished 10 minutes after the treatment.

A 48-year-old woman came into the office with a chief complaint of one week of severe vertigo. Upon questioning her, it was discovered that for the past week she had been substituting a particular artificial sweetener for the sugar in her coffee. Upon clearing her allergy for that particular sugar substitute the vertigo left her.

Still another patient, a 52-year-old male, came in with severe sciatica, with radiation of pain and numbness going down the left leg to the side of the foot. Upon questioning him, it was found that he had been using a large helping of home-made diet orange marmalade for the last couple of weeks. His wife had used another sugar substitute as the sweetener in the marmalade. When the problem was pinned down, he was repeatedly treated by NAET for this sugar substitute. He finally responded to treatment, after four hours of hard work. At the end of this time he was free of his sciatica pain.

A 68-year-old lady was diagnosed as having "Lupus Erythematosus and arthritis." Her white blood cell count dropped as low as 2,000/cubic millimeter. She was advised to get a blood transfusion. During her initial visit in our office, she said that she was taking 6 to 8 grams of vitamin C daily for the past six months. Upon questioning her further, it was discovered that her joint pains had begun six months ago and that the blood count drop was discovered only two months ago. She was found to be highly allergic to vitamin C. She was treated for vitamin C. Ten days after she finished the treatment for vitamin C, she was tested for white blood cell count and her count had gone up to 7,000/cm, which was normal.

A 67-year-old man came to our office with complaints of excruciating pain and red rashes on the lateral parts of the thigh, leg and foot for more than a week. He had seen a few professionals for this problem without any result. His pain and immobility kept increasing. Kinesiological exams focused an allergy to sardines which he had eaten a week ago. He was treated for sardines by NAET, and his pain and rashes disappeared in a few hours.

A 59-year-old woman with a history of vitiligo (white spots all over the body, some under the chin, in front of the ears, leg, back of the neck) for almost 30 years. She was found to be allergic to wool, vitamin C, dust mites, yeast, molds, fruits, yogurt, vinegar, chlorophyll, whole grains and melanin. When she was treated for these items, her white spots were replaced by normal skin pigments.

A 46-year-old man had a peculiar complaint for seven months. He had severe pain on the right forearm, mainly at the wrist joint, for seven months. His right forearm appeared less than half the size of the left forearm. He was under the care of an orthopedic surgeon. He was diagnosed as having carpal tunnel syndrome. The surgeon suggested surgery to release the tension of the median nerve and hoped this would solve the problem. Fortunately, the doctor had a family emergency, and he had to leave the state for two months.

The man was advised to see us by one of his clients, who was one of our pioneer patients, who had experienced relief of an unusual pain disorder four years earlier. He was very desperate at that time and came to our office immediately. Kinesiological testing revealed that he was suffering from an allergy to an artichoke he had eaten seven months ago. He was treated for the artichoke. In less than five minutes his pain was relieved and his forearm returned to normalcy. Forty-eight hours after he was again seen in our office, and he remained free of all the previous symptoms. His carpal tunnel symptoms were caused by the allergy to artichoke. His arm length returned to normal. His pain and discomfort disappeared completely. Of course, he did not have the scheduled surgery for the forearm.

A 38-year-old woman had a history of repeated ovarian cysts and uterine fibroids. She was a vegetarian, and her diet consisted all types of dried beans. She was found to be very allergic to beans or vegetable proteins. Treatment was given for all types of beans. A month after the completion of the treatment, she began having profuse white vaginal discharge, which lasted for two months. After six months, a gynecological exam and an ultra sound treatment showed no trace of fibroid or cysts. Four years after the treatments, she could enjoy all her bean dishes yet still remained free of cysts or tumors.

A 24-year-old girl came in complaining of bilateral breast abscesses over a period of three days. She had severe pain and could not wear normal cloths due to swelling and pain. She had eaten potatoes four days in a row before she developed the pain and swelling of the breast. She was treated for potato by NAET immediately. She felt 60% better soon after the treatment. She needed two more treatments and at the end of two days her breasts became normal. Amazingly, the body healed itself by disposing of the redness, abscess-filled boils, and the painful abscess.

A 36-year-old woman was introduced to a new light, alcoholic cocktail that consisted of grapefruit, Irish whiskey and tequila.

She drank this cocktail every night for three nights in a row. The fourth morning she woke up with a severe pain in her left ovary. She saw her gynecologist and got the terrible news that she had a large mass in the left ovary. Concerned, the gynecologist sent her for an ultrasound examination. She had an orange sized cyst in the left ovary. She was advised by the group of doctors to have surgery immediately to prevent pain and rupture of the cyst. She was sent to the emergency room.

This girl was one of our patients who had previously been treated for various allergic reactions in our office. She was surprised by the news of the cyst and the possible surgery. Her husband was away on a business trip. Nervous and frightened, she remembered to call me to ask my opinion about the situation. From the series of questions she answered, the cause of the sudden appearance of the cyst was pinpointed to the alcoholic cocktails she drank three nights in a row.

She was asked to come to our office with the cocktail. She was treated by NAET for the allergy to the drink and was given acupuncture to reduce the pain and discomfort. She complained of nausea, dizziness, and excruciating pain on the left lower quadrant of the abdomen. The acupuncture points and methods used for the treatment were Spleen - 6, Pericardium - 6, with tonification, Large Intestine - 3, bilateral and "ashi" points with the reduction method. Within 40 minutes of the treatment, her pain was reduced to "1" on the scale of 1 - 10. She was treated everyday with acupuncture for the next three days. Then an ultrasound test was repeated. All of the tests performed on her were negative for any cysts.

A 13-year-old boy was brought to the office at approximately 2:00 p.m. with severe pain in the right lower quadrant of the abdomen which had persisted for 45 minutes. His pain was "10" on the scale of 1 - 10. He complained of nausea and had a body temperature of 100.8 degrees Fahrenheit, by mouth. His right lower abdomen was very tender to touch. His white blood cell count was 10,900/cm. He demonstrated all the signs of an inflamed appendix.

Kinesiological examination revealed that he was allergic to the Rice Krispies treats he had eaten at a friend's house for lunch about 11.00 a.m. the same day. His friend's house was 40 miles from the clinic and to get the exact sample of the Rice Krispies treat for NAET treatment was not practical. By then he threw up on the bed. We collected the vomit in a glass bottle, and he was found to be very allergic to the vomit. He was instantly treated for the vomit by NAET. Within 20 minutes after the treatment, his pain reduced to "2" on the scale of 1 - 10. We had to repeat the treatments four times in 50 minutes. After the fourth treatment, he had no pain, no nausea and smiled first time in hours.

Food coloring causes many allergies among people. A 42-year-old female patient suffered from severe persistent perspiration on her palms, feet, axilla and groin. After careful observation, it was found that she had perspired profusely soon after she ate some lemon colored candies. She got relief from her problem after she was treated for her allergy to yellow food-coloring.

Sulfites are another widely publicized substance that was added to salads and potato in the fast food industry and at restaurant salad bars as a preservative. The intention was to maintain freshness, or at least the appearance of freshness and flavor, as these vegetables sat out in display cases for long periods of time. Unfortunately for some asthma sufferers, sulfites are salt derivatives of sulfuric acid. Many asthma sufferers are highly allergic to sulfur.

A 65-year-old female patient went to a restaurant and ate taquitos. The guacamole sauce was very tart. She took the leftovers home for dinner. A couple of hours after eating, she suffered a severe asthmatic attack. Later, it was discovered that the sulfite, added to the guacamole sauce to preserve its beautiful green color, triggered her asthmatic attack. The use of sulfites in foods is banned in California, but it is legal to use "whiten-all," which acts just like sulfites and also causes many allergic reactions, especially in asthma sufferers.

A male patient, age 51, woke up with a severe toothache in the first upper molar. His dentist was out of town so he decided to try to assuage the pain by acupuncture, until his dentist returned. Upon questioning him in our office, it was discovered that he had eaten a Mexican dinner with guacamole the night before he woke up with the toothache. He was treated for sulfites, and in a few minutes his toothache subsided. The next day, at our insistence, he visited the dentist and was told his tooth was in perfect condition.

Homogenized milk causes concern to a lot of patients in the United States. Even after they clear for the milk allergy, homogenized milk drinkers face some allergic reaction once in a while. This depends mainly on cattle feed. It was found out from various dairies that they have no control over what the cows are fed every day. Most of the nut-oil companies, after extracting the oils, dry the leftovers into compact cakes and sell them to the dairies. In the dairies, these cakes are randomly fed to the cows. When the cows secrete milk, some of the substances from the nuts are also secreted through the milk. Sometimes, if the cows are fed with hay and grasses that are sprayed with pesticides, these substances are also excreted in the milk. When an allergic person drinks this milk, they can react at any time. This particular reaction is not due to any allergy to milk but to the pesticides or other ingredients in the milk sample. This should be kept in mind when treating for milk allergy.

Great care must be taken, as can be seen from the above-listed cases, to know exactly what is contained in each and every thing a person with allergies puts into his mouth. If everyone could get proficient in muscle-response testing, most hazardous accidents from food allergies could be prevented by testing before eating the foods.

CONTACTANTS

Contactants produce their effect by direct contact with the skin. They include the well-known poison oak, poison ivy, poison sumac, cats, dogs, rabbits, cosmetics, soaps, skin cremes, detergents, rubbing alcohol, gloves, hair dyes, various types of plant oils, chemicals such as gasoline, dyes, acrylic nails, nail polish, fabrics, formaldehyde, etc.

Allergic reactions to contactants can be different in each person, and may include asthma, skin rashes, hives, fainting spells, migraine headaches, cough, joint pains, various kinds of arthritis, stomachaches, constipation, mental confusion, swelling of the body, frequent urination, mental irritability, insomnia, skin cancer, etc. It is apparent that something contacted by the skin can produce symptoms as devastating to the patient as anything ingested or inhaled.

A 44-year-old female school teacher suffered from a severe hacking, dry cough for 18 months. She tried various prescription medicines to stop cough, with no result. She coughed 24 hours a day. She could hardly sleep during the night. She was frustrated, and her family was frustrated with this unsolved problem. She was tested by an allergist and found to be allergic to dusts, insects, grasses, and pollens. She was treated for most of the food, fabrics, dusts, grasses, pollens and chemicals in her environment, with out any positive results. Finally, she was found to be allergic to her acrylic nails.

Upon questioning her further, it was discovered that 18 months ago she started using the acrylic nails to cover up her brittle nails. She was asked to remove the nails for a day just to see if that made any difference in her cough. To her amazement, she stopped coughing completely as soon as she removed the nails and put away. The next day she was treated for the nails and her 18 month cough was gone.

A 23-year-old woman suffered from a type of dermatitis that did not respond to the treatments of food products, chemicals or environmental items. Various parts of her body such as neck, lips, face, chest etc., showed dry, cracked furrows with clear water, filled blisters which looked like first degree burns. Often she had blood and serum oozing from weeping blisters. History revealed that she was alright until she moved in with her fiance, a year and half ago. She was allergic to her fiance's saliva. Her mysterious problem was solved when she was treated for his saliva by NAET.

A 27-year-old man was allergic to his dog. He suffered from asthma and upper respiratory problems. He was treated for the dog hair and danders, but the allergy did not improve. Later when he was treated for the dog's saliva, his allergy was cleared.

A 38-year-old man had depression for most of his life. He had tried various treatments, including psychotherapy. He was found to be allergic to iron. He had wrought-iron ornamental works all over his house. When he was treated for iron metal, his depression cleared.

A 24-year-old woman suffered from chronic fatigue syndrome for four years. She suffered from severe brain fog, poor memory, sudden shooting pains in her brain, sharp pains in parts of her body, blurred vision, heart palpitation, excessive hunger, insomnia and severe constipation. She had a stainless steel implant in her knee, which had been implanted after a football accident when she was 16 years old. When she was treated for the stainless steel, her brain fog decreased. Her heartbeats became regular. Her appetite got regulated, sharp shooting pains disappeared, sleep was better and most of her CFS syndromes improved. The allergy to stainless steel was causing most of her unpleasant symptoms.

A female patient, 28 years old, was under treatment for lupus at a lupus clinic. She had severe joint pains most of the time. She suffered from severe insomnia, mental cloudiness, poor memory, mental irritability and debilitating multiple joint pains. She was on three different kinds of analgesics, which she took every three hours, to control her pain. Extremely hot, cold or cloudy weather affected her immensely. On such days, she stayed indoors with pain pills and warm water.

When she was evaluated in our office, she was found to be allergic to all the fabrics she was wearing, however, she was not allergic to any food or drugs. She was treated individually for cotton, polyester, acrylic, nylon, plastics and leather. At the end of the session, it was found that her symptoms of lupus had diminished greatly. Her bodily disturbances with the weather changes also disappeared. She had been visiting the lupus clinic once a month. When she visited the clinic after she cleared her allergies, she showed great improvement in her laboratory blood tests. She was told the best news by her doctor -- that her lupus was in remission. Three years later, she remains absolutely symptom-free.

A 24-year-old patient suffered from a peculiar kind of arthritis. Doctors diagnosed her condition as psychosomatic arthritis and could not prescribe any medicine to help her with her problem. She was very active and worked as a registered nurse in an intensive care unit. On certain days, she complained of severe multiple joint pains, and she had to be absent from work several times. Her whole body got stiff, and certain days, she could not even hold a pen without stiffness and pain in her hands. Her knuckles and wrists became swollen. She was forced to spend the next couple of days in bed with aspirin and water. She suffered from this problem once a week, sure as clockwork, and she used to take as many as 30 aspirin a day!

When she was evaluated, it was revealed that she was making homemade bread with wheat flour for her husband once a week. She never liked wheat products, so she never ate them. She used to knead the dough with her hands. She was highly allergic to wheat and contact with the dough was the cause of her once-a-week arthritis pain.

Another woman, age 39, suffered from severe insomnia. She was using a well known brand of face and body cream at night. It was found that she was highly allergic to this cream, which was the cause of her insomnia.

An infant was one week old when his mother found him one day in his crib without any signs of life. He wasn't breathing. She grabbed him and shook him. Her husband called the paramedics. Within three minutes, paramedics arrived and found his heart had stopped. They used a defibrillator and revived him. John was alive once again, his breathing and heart beat restored.

He was taken to the hospital for monitoring for 48 hours, after which he was sent home with a beeping monitor. Whenever he stopped breathing, the beeper went off. Back home his beeper was going on frequently, at least five to eight times a day. His mother, grandmother and father watched closely for 24 hours. Although he was doing fine at the hospital, he was having breathing stoppages frequently at home. Later on, it was found that he was allergic to the fancy, attractive, plastic crib covering and other plastic accessories. After he was treated for these plastic items by Nambudripad's Allergy Elimination Techniques, he did not have the problems again.

Another woman, age 49, suffered from chronic asthma and nasal polyps. She worked as an interior decorator and was on disability for seven years due to these problems. When she was evaluated in our office, she was found to be allergic to formaldehyde, one of the ingredients in hundreds of substances around her. It is found in fabrics, name tags on dresses, pressed woods, inks, white-outs, leather goods, plastics, finishing materials in many items, decaffeinated coffee, ice cream, etc., as well as embalming fluid. Her asthma became controlled when she was successfully treated for formaldehyde.

A 72-year-old woman complained of frequent urination for ten years or so. She was forced to get up at least five to six times each night. She could not get continuous sleep, which made her very tired. She was seen and examined by a couple of urologists and given a few antibiotics for possible bladder infections. Nothing worked in her case. She also started waking up with severe headaches in the mornings. She was in an extreme neurotic condition when she was evaluated in our office. The woman was found to be highly allergic to cotton. The use of cotton under garments gave her constant bladder irritation, frequent urination and mimicked bladder infection. Her nephew had given her a cotton night dress a year earlier for her birthday. Whenever she slept in that nightshirt, she experienced fainting spells or woke up with migraine headaches. After she was treated for cotton by Nambudripad's Allergy Elimination Techniques, she was able to overcome her problems permanently.

Woolens may also cause allergies. We have seen people who cannot wear wool without breaking out in rashes. Some people who are sensitive to wool, also react to creams with lanolin base, since lanolin is derived from sheep wool. Some people can be allergic to cotton socks, orlon socks, or woolen socks with symptoms of knee pain, etc. People can also be allergic to carpets and drapes that could cause knee pains and joint pains.

A 44-year-old male patient was seen in our office for long-standing athletes foot. He was a tennis player and would generally wear tennis socks and shoes. After a heavy session of tennis, he would come home limping from knee pain. He associated the pain with increasing age and possible arthritis. After evaluation, it was discovered that he was highly allergic to the particular tennis socks he wore. After the treatments for the socks, his knee pains were gradually relieved, and his athlete's foot disappeared.

A 14-year-old soccer player hurt and sprained his ankles very frequently. The cause of his frequent falls was his orlon/ cotton socks and canvas shoes. After he received treatment for the socks and shoes, he did not sprain his ankle again, at least until he finished high school. The chemicals used in tennis shoes, mercaptobenzothiazole (MBT) and dibenzothiazyl (DBTD) are allergens to many people and known to cause cancer in rats.

A pharmacist suffered from allergy-induced athlete's foot for years because of a common prescription to keep the foot dry, medicated, and wear cotton socks. He was allergic to his socks.

We had a few other female patients who were allergic to their panty hose and suffered from leg cramps, swollen legs, psoriasis, and persistent yeast infections. Toilet paper and paper towels also cause problems, mimicking yeast infections in many people.

A 38-year-old woman went to see a circus and she used their temporary rest rooms. In a few minutes she began itching and burning in her private areas, mimicking a yeast infection. She quickly remembered the toilet paper and brought a piece to the office the next morning. She was allergic to it. Her discomfort ceased soon after she was treated for the toilet paper by Nambudripad's Allergy Elimination Techniques.

Many people are allergic to crude oils and their derivatives, which include plastic and synthetic rubber products. Can you imagine the difficulty of living life in this modern society, trying to be completely free from products made of crude oil? A person would literally be immobilized. The phones we use, the naugahyde chairs we sit on, the milk containers we use, the polyester fabrics we wear, most of the face and body creams we use, all are made from a common product - crude oil!

One of the secretaries in our office was attending a computer demonstration. Five minutes after the demonstration began, she complained of feeling hot all over her body and uncomfortable. She was working at the computer keyboard. Instantly, she began having blisters on her lips, rashes on her face and sensation of light-headedness. The author found that the keyboard (plastic) material was causing the problem. She was treated for the special plastic keyboard and sent home. The next day, when she returned to work, she felt fine and ever since she has worked on that computer keyboard without any further ill effects.

Food items, normally classified as ingestants, may also act as a contactant on persons who handle them constantly over time.

A 59-year-old male baker came in with severe skin rashes and itching of both hands and arms below the elbow. Cortisone cream kept his itching and weeping ulcers under control. He worked four days a week, Thursday through Sunday. By Sunday, his skin became raw and weeping. The next three days he used Cortisone cream, and by Thursday his skin looked better. This had been going on for 27 years when he came to us and was evaluated. He was found to be highly allergic to wheat flour, which he contacted all day, every day of his working life as a baker.

Other career-produced allergies have been diagnosed for cooks, waiters, grocery-store keepers, clerks, gardeners, etc. Virtually no trade or skill is exempt from contracting allergens.

A 49-year-old man complained of severe pains in the right elbow, the wrist joint and the first interphalangeal joints. He was treated for a carpel tunnel syndrome, tenosynovitis, and tennis elbow many times before he came to our office. When he was evaluated in our office, he was found to be highly allergic to paper, one of the tools of his trade as a writer.

Another example of a paper allergy was observed during an interview with an attorney, who complained that he always came away from his office with a headache and feeling so tired that he could only go home and immediately go to bed. This attorney was allergic to paper, with a completely different reaction from that of the writer.

A female piano teacher, with acute asthma, complained of wheezing every time she played the piano. It was discovered she was allergic to the ivory of the keyboard.

A salesman who complained of severe backaches after being on the road for a day was found to be allergic to the acrylic seat covers in the car.

INJECTANTS

Allergens are injected into the skin, muscles, joints and blood vessels in the form of various serums, antitoxins, vaccines and drugs. They also include substances entering the body through insect bites. As in any other allergic reaction, the injection of a sensitive drug into the system runs the risk of producing dangerous allergic reactions. To the sensitive person, the drug actively becomes a poison, with the same effect as an injection of arsenic. No one would intentionally give an injection of a potentially dangerous drug to a person. However, some drugs seem to become more allergenic for certain people over time, without the person being aware of the potential risk. Take the increasing incidents of allergies to the drug penicillin, as an example. The reactions vary from hives to diarrhea to anaphylactic shock and death.

A school teacher, in her mid-30's, had frequent, severe itching and hives for many years. She said her problems started after taking some penicillin injections a few years ago. She was found to be allergic to penicillin and treated by Nambudripad's Allergy Elimination Techniques. Her skin problem diminished dramatically after the penicillin treatment.

Most of us do not often consider an insect bite in the same way as we would an injection received from a physician or a member of his staff, but the result is quite the same. At the point of the bite, a minute amount of the body fluid (saliva) of the insect is injected into the body. These fluids may be incidental to the bite. They may be simply secretions normal to the salivary gland or biting part of the insect, or they may be a necessary part of the biting mechanism, such as the saliva of the mosquito, which is formulated to keep the host's blood from coagulating so blood extraction is not difficult.

These fluids may also be specifically formulated to produce immobilizing pain, in order to protect the insect from its own predators, such as the spider that uses its bite to secure food and inflict pain in the defense of its territory; the bee that uses its sting for defense, and the wasp that uses its sting to obtain food and defend its nest.

Certain animal bites also inject near lethal amounts of toxins into the bloodstream of victims, again to immobilize prey and to protect itself from its own predators, or accidental harm from a clumsy neighbor. Examples include the general classification of pit vipers and one or two lizards. It also includes a number of fish and crustaceans that are capable of inflicting painful stings or puncture-delivered poisons from sharp spines and/or spine-like fins. Bites from mammals also fit into this category. They include bites of children which can produce considerable infection, at the site of the bite, and the injection of the dreaded of dreaded virus from the bite of an infected animal.

The normal reaction to a bite, other than the obvious lethal bites, ranges from mild swelling around the site of the injection, a mild reddening and, of course, a slight to moderate discomfort in the body from attempting to free the toxin that produces itching. Rarely are these bites and stings lethal to the normally insensitive person.

For some people, however, a sting or a bite by an animal or insect is potentially lethal. Even a single mosquito bite may produce an extreme and sudden onset of edema (the abnormal collection of fluids in the body tissue and cells) and severe respiratory distress. There have been many cases of anaphylactic shock, respiratory and/or cardiac failure in sensitive persons, following the slightest insect bite.

A female patient of 59 came to the office with a typical case of accidental serum injection poisoning. She was vacationing in London where she was stung by a bee, while boarding a bus. Although she had known that she reacted strongly to insect bites as a child, she had no idea how much the allergic condition had increased over the years. Within minutes she was feeling nausea and light-headedness, and was having difficulty breathing. Luckily, she was transported to a hospital emergency care unit. By the time she reached the hospital, she experienced some respiratory distress. She was treated by the doctors and hospitalized for three days.

Upon returning to the United States ten days later, she was still experiencing some cellulitis in her left arm and was brought to our office. Soon after she received treatments by Nambudripad's Allergy Elimination Techniques to desensitize for bee sting, her cellulitis of the arm diminished. One year later, when she was camping, she was stung by bees again. This time she panicked and her friends drove her to the nearest hospital about 40 miles away. She did not have any unpleasant reactions. They sat in the hospital parking lot and waited for two long hours to see whether she was going to have any reactions. Since she felt alright, they returned without entering the hospital. The next day she was seen in our office. She had many bee sting marks on her arms, which looked like mild prickly heat.

A 79-year-old male patient from North Carolina worked as a painter in his young days and had been stung by wasps many times, while he was on the ladder painting houses. He developed cancer, which had metastasized throughout his body by the time it was discovered. He was given six months to live. He refused any traditional treatment for his problem but was treated for various allergies, one of which was wasp stings. Soon his condition began to change. His energy level picked up, his appetite increased, and he did not feel sleepy or fatigued any more. He increased his activities and started playing golf once again.

A year later, when he went to the same clinic that had given him six months to live, his doctors were amazed at his condition. "Some miracle has happened," they said. "Somehow your cancer has gone into remission." Actually, it was the repeated injection of wasp venom into his body that created the cancer. An abnormal proliferation of the cells in his body was the reaction he experienced from the wasp stings. He did not show any external reactions such as hives or swelling, etc. When he was treated for the same toxin, his body responded well and created the antidote to destroy the wasp venom and the carcinoma that was the side effect of the wasp stings.

Many carcinomas result from some type of allergies; if one could but trace the particular allergen, the most serious disease of mankind might be cured. Good detective work is essential to find the basic root of the problem.

INFECTANTS

Infectants are allergens that produce their effect by causing a sensitivity to an infectious agent, such as bacteria. For example, when tuberculin bacteria is introduced as part of a diagnostic test to determine a patient's sensitivity or reaction to that particular agent, an allergic reaction may result. This may occur during skin patch, or scratch tests done in the normal course of allergy testing in traditional Western medical circles.

Infectants differ from injectants as allergens because of the nature of the allergic substances; that is, the substance is a known injectant and is limited in the amount administered to the patient. A slight prick of the skin introduces the toxin through the epidermis and a pox or similar harmless skin lesion will erupt, if the patient is allergic or reactive to that substance. For most people, the pox soon dries up and forms a scab which eventually drops off, without much discomfort. However, for those individuals who are reactive to these tests, it is not uncommon to experience fainting, nausea, fever, swelling (not only at the scratch site but over the whole body), respiratory distress, etc.

In other words, the introduction of an allergen into the reactive person's system runs the potential risk of causing a severe reaction, regardless of the reason or the amount of the toxic substance used. Great care must be taken in the administration of tests that are designed to produce an allergic reaction.

Various vaccinations and immunizations may also produce such allergic reactions. Some children after they receive their usual immunization get very sick physically and emotionally. Such was the case of a 4 year old boy who became very sick after a regular DPT immunization. He had continuous fever (102 degrees Fahrenheit) for six weeks. Finally, when the fever came down to a normal level, he had a dull response to every day activities. He became normal after he was treated for DPT.

A 46-year-old woman had complained of severe sinusitis and respiratory problems, including asthma, for 28 years. She was admitted to the hospital and given Cortisone injections when she was 18 years old. She almost went into shock at that time and finally recovered from the episode. Soon after she came out of the hospital, she began experiencing severe sinus problems and upper respiratory problems. At age 46, when she was treated for Cortisone, she reacted violently. When she successfully completed the treatment for the Cortisone, her 28 year old upper respiratory problems got better.

It should be noted that bacteria, viruses, etc., are contacted in numerous ways. Our casual contact with objects and people exposes us daily to dangerous contaminants and possible illnesses. When our autoimmune systems are functioning properly, we pass off the illness without notice. When our systems are not working at maximum performance levels, we experience infections, fevers, etc.

From a strictly allergenic standpoint, however, contact with an injectant does not produce the expected reaction for that particular injectant; rather a more typical allergic reaction takes place, as can be seen in the tuberculin test. It is clear that the reaction to the test was not a case of tuberculosis but rather a mild allergic response that resulted in an infectious eruption under the skin.

A 36-year-old woman had multiple sclerosis for the past 12 years. Her symptoms began after giving birth to her child by cesarean section. During her child birth, she was injected with spinal anesthesia. She was found to be highly allergic to the spinal anesthesia that was used 12 years ago. Her symptoms got better when she was cleared for the allergy to the anesthesia.

A 26-year-old woman was found to have had multiple sclerosis for the last five years. When she came to our office, she was unable to walk with out assistance, and she was almost blind in both eyes. In her case, her silicone breast implant was the cause. When she was cleared for the silicone implant her symptoms got better. Her sight regained, she became steady on her feet, was able to pass the driver's license test and was able to drive again.

PHYSICAL AGENTS

Heat, cold, sunlight, dampness, drafts or mechanical irritants may also cause allergic reactions and are known as physical allergens. When the patient suffers from more than one allergy, physical agents can affect the patient greatly. If the patient has already eaten some allergic food item, then walks in cold air or drafts, he might develop upper respiratory problems, sore throat, asthma or joint pains, etc., depending on his tendency toward health problems.

Some people are very sensitive to cold or heat, whether they have eaten any allergic food or not. Such cases are very rare. One of the young patients who came to our office had a history of canker sores whenever he walked in the sun. He was highly allergic to vitamin D, one of the vitamins produced in the body with the help of sunlight. After he was treated by Nambudripad's Allergy Elimination Techniques for vitamin D, the incidents of canker sores, as a result of walking in the sun, diminished.

A 74-year-old woman liked to drink cold water, but she always choked on icy cold water. She also developed an allergic dry cough whenever she ate ice cream. She was treated for all the ingredients in the ice cream, yet her coughing spells and choking incidents persisted. She was finally treated for actual ice cubes. Afterwards, she could enjoy ice water and ice cream without choking.

A 42-year-old woman became very disturbed mentally and physically whenever it was hot. Her whole body swelled up in the hot season or if she walked in the sun for a few minutes. She could never drink hot liquids or eat hot foods without getting sick. Whenever she ate hot foods, she would have a paroxysmal tachycardia (very speedy heart rate) and her whole body would turn red and swollen. She was treated for very hot water. A few minutes after treatment by Nambudripad's Allergy Elimination Techniques, she had severe abdominal cramps and severe continuous diarrhea. When she was successfully treated for hot water, her body began to adjust to the heat in a normal way.

A week after the treatment, there was a heat wave in Southern California. The temperatures reached 104 degrees. Her car broke down mid-afternoon, and she had to walk for about 15 minutes to reach the gas station for help. Amazingly, she did not react to the heat as she would have before the treatment. She did not even have the usual foot swelling. Now she enjoys hot herbal teas and soups, and she lost 35 pounds since the treatment for heat. In her case, the allergy to heat was the cause of her obesity.

A 49-year-old woman had severe hot flashes for the last three years. She was on hormone supplements, but nothing gave her relief from hot flashes. She was found to be allergic to heat, sugar and hormones. After she was cleared for the allergy to the above items, her hot flashes stopped completely.

A woman, 58 years old, suffered from Raynaud's disease. The tip of her fingers remained dark blue on a cold day. She was allergic to cold, citrus fruits, and meat products. She felt better when she was cleared for the above items.

A 67-year-old man used to get severe knee pains on both knees when ever it is cold or cloudy. He was found to be allergic to sodium chloride, potassium, and cold. Probably, when he was surrounded by cold, his sodium-potassium pump became less active. This may have caused poor circulation and water collection in larger joints. This in turn caused the pain during cold weather.

Many arthritic patients, asthma patients, migraine patients, PMS patients, and mental patients have exaggerated symptoms on a cold, cloudy or rainy day. These types of patients could suffer from severe allergy to electrolytes, cold or a combination of both.

Some patients react to heat or cold violently, getting aches and pains during a cloudy day, and icy cold hands and feet even if they are clad in a dozen pairs of warm socks, etc. These patients have hypo-functioning immune systems. When they finish the treatment program, they do not continue to feel cold or get sick with the heat or cold.

In the case of skin cancer, the causative factor may not only be overexposure to the sun, as many people think, but may be due to allergies to sun-tan lotion, skin cream, shaving cream, razor blades (stainless steel), clothing or other allergenic products.

Consistent use of these products may well cause skin irritation or skin cancer.

A man, age 32, who frequently had skin cancer on his face, was evaluated and found to be highly allergic to the stainless steel blade of the razor he used. The use of a popular skin cream was the cause of the beginning of skin cancer in one patient. She was allergic to vitamin A and to the skin cream. After she was treated for these substances, her lesions cleared up.

GENETIC CAUSES

Discovery of possible tendencies toward allergies carried over from parents and grandparents opens a large door to achieving optimum health. Most people inherit the allergic tendency from their parents or grandparents. Allergies can also skip generations and be manifested very differently in parents than in their children.

A 35-year-old female patient had suffered from various allergies since she was an infant. When she was three weeks old, she broke out in a rash, which turned into big heat boils and pustules. Her parents tried various medications in attempts to cure her, including allopathy, homeopathy and herbal medicines.
Finally, herbal medicine brought it under control. She had the outbreaks of skin lesions every now and then until she was ten years old, when she developed a type of severe, debilitating arthritis which continued until she was in her late teens. She then developed migraine headaches and severe insomnia along with arthritis. She tried various medicines from different doctors without much relief.

She was evaluated and found to be reacting to malaria parasites. It was discovered that her mother and father were malaria victims before she was born. The effect of malaria from her parents transferred to her, and was manifested in her body as skin and joint problems (i.e., arthritis). When she was successfully treated for malaria, her health took a quantum leap.

Many people with various allergic manifestations responded well to the treatment of various disease agents that had been transmitted from parents. A woman who suffered from bronchial asthma was cleared of her asthma when she was treated for pneumococcus, the bacterium responsible for pneumonia. Both of her parents had died of pneumonia soon after her birth.

A man of 44 responded well to the treatment for diphtheria, thus clearing his chronic bronchitis. He had inherited the tendency toward allergies from his mother, who almost died from diphtheria when she was seven. The reaction to diphtheria was manifested in him as bronchitis, sinusitis and arthritis.

A 55-year-old woman suffered from the Epstein-Barr virus and various allergies. After treatment for the virus, her response was very encouraging. Upon questioning her, it was found that her Japanese parents, uncles and aunts died of tuberculosis. She was immediately tested and treated for tuberculosis and she became allergy free and healthy once again.

Parents with rheumatic fever may transmit the disease to their offspring, but in the children the rheumatic fever agent did not manifest in its original form.

A woman of 42 had severe migraines all her life. Her mother had rheumatic fever as a child. Treatment for rheumatic fever lessened her migraines.

Carcinomas also can be a result of various allergies, sometimes as offshoots of inherited allergies from parents or as an allergy acquired from one's own life-style. Various chemical agents around us are carcinogenic, but it is better to check out all the possibilities of genetically transmitted allergenic offshoots in cases of cancer, when the cancer does not respond to western traditional treatment.

MOLDS AND FUNGI

Molds and fungi are in a category by themselves, because of the numerous ways that they are contacted as an allergen in everyday life. They can be ingested, inhaled, touched or even, as in the case of Penicillin, injected. They come in the form of airborne spores, making up a large part of the dust we breathe or pick up in our vacuum cleaners; fluids such as our drinking water; as dark fungal growth in the corners of damp rooms; as athlete's foot; and in particularly obnoxious vaginal conditions commonly called "yeast infections." They grow on trees and in the damp soil. They are a source of food, as in truffles and mushrooms; of diseases such as ring worm and the aforementioned yeast infections, and of healing, as in the tremendous benefits mankind has derived from the drug Penicillin.

Reactions to these substances are as varied as other kinds of allergies. This is because they are a part of one of the largest known classifications of biological entities. Because of the number of ways they can be introduced into the human anatomy, the number of reactions are multiplied considerably.

Fungi are parasites that grow on living as well as decaying organic matter. That means some forms are found growing in the human anatomy. The problem of athlete's foot is a prime example.

Athlete's foot is a human parasite fungus that grows anywhere in the body, where the area is fairly moist and not exposed to sunlight or air. It is particularly difficult to eliminate, and treatment generally consists of a topical preparation, multiple daily cleansing of the area, a medicinal powder, and wearing light cotton socks to avoid further infection from dyes used in colored wearing apparel.

It is contracted by contact with the fungus and is often passed from person to person anywhere there is the potential for contact (i.e., gymnasium, shower, locker rooms and other areas where people share facilities and walk barefoot). Thus, the name athlete's foot. If it is a real athlete's foot, it will clear with the Nambudripad's Allergy Elimination Techniques treatment, but certain allergies, like allergies to socks made of cotton, orlon, or nylon, etc., can mimic athlete's foot. In such cases, athlete's foot may not clear by using medications.

A 31-year-old man came to the clinic for treatment of athlete's foot. In the interview he disclosed that he had suffered from athlete's foot for years. Everything he tried was without success. The infection not only was distracting and painful but also was destroying the toe nails. The problem was getting so bad that it started to interfere with his passion for tennis. During testing for allergies, it was discovered that he was allergic to cotton and had been using cotton socks all the time. He also mentioned that he washed his feet in a special preparation three times daily and dried them with cotton towels. After treatment for cotton, his athlete's foot also cleared up.

Allergies to cotton, orlon, nylon, or paper could result in the explosions of infections including Ascomycetes fungi (yeast) that women are finding so troublesome. Feminine tampons, toilet papers, douches, and deodorants also cause yeast infections.

CHAPTER THREE

DIAGNOSIS OF ALLERGIES

Allergic conditions occur much more frequently than is realized, except by those who have made a special study of this condition and, of course, by sufferers of serious allergic reactions. Every year there are more and more recognized cases of allergies in the United States. Statistics show that at least 50 percent of the population suffers from a more or less acute form of allergy. Most people will be interested in the methods of diagnosis in traditional Western medicine, as well as in the oriental medicine; some of the common treatments in both; the chances of recovery; and the probable length of time treatments take. Since the purpose of this book is to provide information about the new treatment method of Nambudripad's Allergy Elimination Techniques, more attention will be given to Oriental medicine.

More than in other diseases, it is extremely important for the patient to cooperate with the physician in order to obtain the best results. It is the author's hope that this chapter will help bring about a clearer understanding between allergists and their patients because, in order to obtain the most satisfactory results, the allergists and patients must work together as a team.

The first step in diagnosing an allergy, for the allergist, is to take a thorough history of the patient which should include, among other things, a record of any allergic symptoms in the patient's family. The patient will be asked whether either of his or her parents suffers from asthma or hay fever, has ever had hives, reacted to a serum injection (such as tetanus antitoxin, DPT), or had any other type of skin trouble. Additionally they will be asked whether they were unable to eat certain foods, complained of sinusitis, runny nose, frequent colds or flu, had dyspepsia or indigestion, ever suffered from acute indigestion or a number of other conditions that might have had an allergic cause or where an allergy may have been a contributing factor although not recognized as such at the time.

These questions will be asked not only with regard to the patient, but also to other relatives, such as grandparents, aunts, uncles, brothers, sisters and cousins. This is because an allergic tendency is not always inherited directly from the parents. It may skip generations or be manifested in nieces or nephews rather than in direct descendants.

The careful allergist will also determine whether or not such diseases as tuberculosis, cancer, diabetes, rheumatic or glandular disorders exist in the patient's family history. All of these facts help give the allergist a more complete picture of the hereditary characteristics of the patient. Allergic tendency is inherited. It may be manifested differently in different people. An actual allergic condition such as asthma may not be inherited. Parents may have had cancer or rheumatism and the child manifested that allergic inheritance as asthma.

When the family history has been completed, the allergist will probably require a look into the history of the patient's allergic attacks. "When did your first attack occur?" should be his or her first question. "Did your allergy first occur when you were an infant/child, or did you first notice the symptoms after you were full grown?" When a careful history has been taken, it will often be discovered, sometimes to the patient's own surprise, that his or her first symptoms occurred in early childhood. He or she may have suffered from infantile eczema but never associated it with the asthma that did not appear until middle age.

Next, the doctor will want to know the circumstances surrounding, and immediately preceding, the first symptoms. His or her questions will probably be, "Did you change your diet or go on a special diet? Did you eat something new that you haven't eaten lately, say for about two or three months? Did you eat one type of food repeatedly, everyday for a few days? Did the symptoms follow a childhood illness such as whooping cough, measles, chickenpox, diphtheria, or any immunization for such an illness? Did they follow some other illness such as influenza, pneumonia, or a major operation? Did the symptoms first appear at adolescence or after you had a baby? Were they first noticed after you acquired a cat, a dog or even a bird? Did they appear after an automobile accident or any such major physical or mental trauma? Did they appear after a lengthy exposure to the sun, such as a day at the beach or 36 holes of golf?"

Any one of these things may be responsible for triggering a severe allergic manifestation or may precipitate the first noticeable symptoms of an allergic condition. Therefore, it is very important these questions be answered as fully and accurately as possible so that the allergist can get a complete history of the allergies.

Other important questions relate to the frequency of attacks and when they occur. If the symptoms occur only at specific times of the year, it is very likely that most of the trouble is due to pollens, although foods may be a factor. Often a patient is sensitive to certain foods but has a natural tolerance that prevents his getting sick until the pollen sensitivity adds sufficient allergens to throw the body into an imbalance. If symptoms occur only on specific days of the week, they are probably due to something that is contacted or eaten on that particular day.

Regular weekly attacks of sneezing and nasal allergy were caused in one patient after she read the Sunday newspaper, the ink of which caused severe allergic reaction. Another patient reacted similarly to the comic section of the newspaper and another man always had a gastrointestinal allergy attack on Sunday morning, the cause of which was traced to a traditional pizza on saturday night with his family. He was allergic to the tomato sauce in the pizza. Still another patient had an allergic attack of sneezing and runny nose on Saturday, which was traced to the chemical compounds of a lotion used to set her hair on Friday afternoon.

The time of day when the attacks occur is also of importance in determining the cause of an allergic manifestation. If it always occurs at night, it is quite likely that there is something in the bedroom that is aggravating the condition. It may be that the patient is sensitive to the feathers in the pillow or comforter, or there may be shrubs, trees, or grasses outside the window which are causing the troubles.

A 38-year-old woman continued to have asthmatic attacks when in bed, although she had been treated successfully for pillows, mattress, fabrics, etc. Finally, it was determined that the rosewood bedroom set and the chest of drawers were the culprits. After she was treated for Rosewood, she no longer had attacks of asthma in her bedroom.

A man, age 42, came with a throat irritation and cough that always started at 4 p.m. and subsided by 8 p.m. He worked as a travel agent and his busy hours were 4-6 p.m. His irritating cough made him very uncomfortable. After proper evaluation, it was discovered that he ate a certain brand of chocolate candy bar every day at 2 p.m. during his break time. By 4 p.m., the allergic reaction from the candy bar showed up in coughing spells. After treatment for chocolate, he did not have the problem again.

Many patients react violently to house dust, different types of furniture, polishes, house plants, water, tap water, and purified water. Most of the city water supplies change the water chemicals once or twice a year. This is done with good intention, however, people with chemical allergies can get sicker if they use the same chemicals over and over for months or years.

Say Good-bye to Illness

Changing the chemicals every now and then gives a change of allergens to the allergic patients and a chance to recover from the existing reactions. This way repeated use of same chemicals can be avoided.

Drinking water comes from different sources. The major sources are ground water and surface water. The ground water supply includes underground aquifers, wells and springs. Most aquifers get their water supply from surface water, which includes lakes, ponds and rivers. Both sources are contaminated by dumping contaminants on to soil. They are carried either throughout the soil to the underground source of water, such as wells and springs, or through the run off of the contaminated soil into lakes and rivers.

Contamination is also caused by natural degradation of vegetation or animal matter and by pollutants carried by air and rain. Surface water is also contaminated by direct dumping into lakes, rivers, and ponds of pollutants like accidental spills, pesticides, septic tank cesspools, landfills, dump or refuse spill, waste lagoon pit or pond, gasoline or diesel spills, industrial disposals, bacteria, virus, parasites such as roundworms, hookworms and tapeworms.

Chlorination is used as the primary disinfectant in water systems across the United States. Chlorination will kill most of the bacteria, but viruses do not get destroyed by any of these cleansing process. Trihalomethanes are also used in cleansing the water, which is a byproduct of chlorine. Ozone is also used as a disinfectant, especially for drinking water. Some of these chemicals are known to cause cancer, birth defects, nervous system disorders, damage to body organs and many other irreversible damages to the consumer's body.

The amount and strength of the pollutants and disinfectants vary in the water. After a heavy rain or flood, pollutants will get mixed with the water in many folds. After the first heavy rain, we usually see an epidemic of influenza all over the country.

A woman, age 54, had complained of having frequent dizzy spells and light-headedness for the last four years. Certain days she had the dizzy spells six or seven times. She had severe joint pains. She complained of tingling sensation all over her body. Certain times she felt extreme fatigue, suffered from severe insomnia, and often got migraine headaches. She was examined by many specialists, had every part of her body x-rayed several times, underwent CAT scans and MRIs of the brain, head and neck. Psychiatric evaluations also were done on her. She was given hormone supplements, iron supplements, but nothing gave her any relief of her symptoms. She had spent thousands of dollars by then, even though most of it was paid by her insurance company.

Finally, she was referred to our office. Her history did not reveal anything significant. Kinesiological tests revealed that her entire problem was caused from some thing she was drinking everyday. Upon questioning her further, it was revealed that she had installed a particular kind of water filter four years ago throughout the house. She was very allergic to the chemical in the filter. She used the filtered water for drinking, washing and bathing. She was advised to disconnect the filter system for a while. As soon as she did so she felt better. Her symptoms did not completely go away until she was treated for that chemical with NAET. Later on , she said that she was too afraid to use the filter system, and she did not use it again. Two years later, before this book was written, she was contacted and she was still in excellent health without any trace of her previous problems.

An 11-year-old girl had severe postnasal drip and sinusitis for two years. Her family also had a water filter installed two years ago. She was treated for the water chemicals and her problem was eliminated. She was still using the same filter system with out any adverse affect one year after treatment.

A 48-year-old woman had a chronic cough since three years, especially at night. She drank two glasses of tap water every night before she went to bed and was found to be allergic to tap water.

A 56-year-old female suffered from asthma for seven years. Whenever she went to bed, she woke up with asthma in couple of hours. Then she would sit up and wheeze for a while, go back to sleep, only to wake up and wheeze again in two more hours. She was told by her doctors that she suffered from cardiac asthma. She was found to be allergic to water. When she was treated for tap water by NAET, her cardiac asthma left her. Upon questioning her further, it was discovered that she had bought this water bed seven years ago. For the past four years she hasn't had another asthmatic episode.

Allergy to corn is one of today's most common allergies, especially in asthmatic and arthritic patients. Cornstarch is found in almost every prepared food. Chinese food contains a lot of it as well as baking soda, baking powder and toothpaste. It is the binding product in almost all pills and vitamins, including aspirin, and Tylenol. Corn syrup is the natural sweetener in almost all the products we see, including soft drinks. Cornsilk is seen in many make-up items. Corn oil is used as vegetable oils.

Another common ingredient in many preparations are the various gums such as acacia gums, karaya gum, etc. Various gums are used in candy bars, yogurt, cream cheese, soft drinks, sauces like soy sauce and barbecue sauce, fast food products, macaroni and cheese, etc. Some people react severely to these gums.

A 43-year-old woman came in with severe pain in her right breast. She had a history of repeated breast abscesses including episodes of being incised and drained seven times during the last two years. She was on antibiotics throughout the year. When questioned, it was revealed that the present problem started after she ate a piece of cheesecake. When the ingredients were examined, it was discovered that the cream cheese that was one of the major ingredients in her recipe had gum as an ingredient. It was revealed that she was consuming a lot of gum in various forms every day. After she was treated for gum, her breast abscess did not return for the next 18 months and probably never will.

Carob is another item that causes many common diseases among allergic people and it is used in almost all health food products. Many health conscious people are turning to natural food products and carob is used as a chocolate and cocoa substitute. It is also used as a natural coloring agent and a natural stiffening agent in soft drinks, cheeses, sauces, etc. One of the causes of "holiday flu" has been found to be allergies mainly to carob, chocolate and turkey.

A 37-year-old woman came to the office during the first week of March with the history of severe excruciating pain under the left breast at the level of the sixth and seventh ribs. Her spleen was enlarged and palpable with severe tenderness. The usual laboratory work showed no abnormality. Upon questioning her in detail, it was discovered that she ate some carob covered cherries during Christmas period. The particular "treat" was presented to her by one of her favorite cousins who came from Europe. She ate about 25 of them in three to four days time. She was a nutrition company distributor and used their protein drink and milk shakes which had carob as flavoring agent. By muscle response testing she was found to be highly reactive to carob. After successful treatment by Nambudripad's Allergy Elimination Techniques she was relieved of her nagging pain.

She was back on the nutrition products without any further discomfort.

After completing the history, allergists should examine the patient for the usual vital signs. A physical examination is performed in regard to any abnormal growth or condition. If the patient has any pain or discomfort, the area of pain in the body should be inspected and recorded for the type of pain, area of pain, and for any relation to an acupuncture point. Most of the time, except for traumas, any pain in the body occurs around some important acupuncture point.

There are 12 major acupuncture meridians in the body. These energy pathways (meridians) are like rivers beginning from the source and flowing through the surface, a long distance to the destination. Many different sized channels and collaterals join the flowing river during its journey. Acupuncture meridians are similar. The starting point of the meridian is usually an end point of a limb, either a hand or foot, which travels a long distance through the body, usually to the other end of the body.

Acupuncture meridians also have various channels and collaterals. Twelve meridians combined with their channels and collaterals cover almost every part of the human body. An acupuncturist is trained to understand the exact location of these pathways of these meridians. For this reason the location of the pain is very important. From this location the acupuncturist will be able to detect which meridian in the energy pathway and which organ in the body are affected. He or she will then be able to predict exactly what the patient's symptoms will be. An acupuncturist will be able to determine what particular allergy could be causing the problem. When the source of the problem is determined, treatment becomes easier.

MUSCLE RESPONSE TEST

Now the patient is ready for the muscle response test(MRT). Various commonly used products can be tested this way to determine the patient's allergy to them. After the muscle response test, the patient is tested on a computerized instrument that is designed to measure the body's electrical conductivity, painlessly at specific electrically sensitive points on the skin, particularly on the hands and feet. The computerized operation is based on two theories that have been shown to be clinically valid.

The first theory comes from mechanics and acupuncture. It was found over 40 years ago that the body's electrical characteristics, measured at specific acupuncture points, are predictive of the health of organs and organ systems along corresponding acupuncture meridians or energy pathways. The computer applies this theory by challenging the body with a very small current and then measuring the body's response. The computer records these measurements to provide data that is helpful in recognizing the intensity and severity of the energy blockage in the body.

The second theory is founded primarily on quantum physics and intelligence. It postulates that the body's functions are controlled and coordinated by a very intelligent part of the body. This intelligent "Master Computer" understands and speaks a number of languages and has the ability to keep track of an incredible amount of information at every moment of the day. The computer, through computer stimulation and other techniques, accesses your master computer and receives bio-feedback information in the form of changes in galvanic skin responses. These changes occur in a meaningful, consistent way, which can be interpreted by your doctor.

The computerized tester is a noninvasive Class III investigational medical device, and, in conjunction with muscle response testing can provide rapid, painless allergy testing and can give a good picture of allergens that affect the body and immune system. Foods, inhalants, epidermals, drugs, chemicals, vitamins, amino acids, pollens, trees, woods, weeds, grasses, molds, fabrics, metals and other materials can be tested for allergies by the computerized tester.

The computerized tester also helps to determine the various intensities of the allergies in degrees on a 0 - 100 scale. This is probably one of the best tests available today to determine allergies. This machine is designed to test food allergies, environmental allergies, chemical allergies, allergies to molds and other fungi, allergies to pollens and trees, allergies to grasses, proteins, vitamins, drugs and phenolics and allergies to radiation, etc. It can be used to test allergies and their intensities before treatment and after treatment, so that we are able to judge and show the body's response to the treatment after each treatment.

This does not involve breaking or puncturing the skin. It does not inflict any pain or discomfort. In a limited amount of time, hundreds of allergies can be tested on the patient. Since the testing probe only touches the skin for a split second for each allergy tested, this can be used for infants and children as well as adults. Another advantage of this machine is that it has a clear screen on which the patient can read his own allergies as they are being recorded. This also produces a printout and stores the data for comparison with the future readings.

There have been many other methods of allergy testing available. Traditional methods of testing have never been very reliable. Western medical allergists generally depend on skin testing such as the scratch test, patch test, etc., in which a very small amount of a suspected allergic substance is introduced into the person's skin through a scratch or an injection. Then the site of injection is observed for any reaction. If there is any reaction at the site of injection, the person is considered to be allergic to that substance. Each item has to be tested in this manner individually. Sometimes certain things can be tested in groups.

There are a few disadvantages to this kind of testing method. Some patients can go into anaphylactic shock due to the introduction of extremely allergic items into the body. It is painful, and, in some cases, the pain and discomfort may last many days. Only one set of allergies can be tested at a time. The patient has to wait for a few days or weeks to get another test, which is also very expensive and not very helpful in identifying allergies to foods and many other substances. Since it is not normal to inject foods under the skin it is not surprising that there shouldn't be much of a reaction when tested like this.

Another prevalent allergy test is called a sublingual test and is used by clinical ecologists and some nutritionists. This involves the installation of a tiny amount of an extract of a test substance under the tongue. If the test is positive, symptoms may appear very rapidly, including dramatic mental and behavioral reactions. Some kinesiologists also test this way. A tiny amount of the food substance is placed under the tongue and an indicator muscle is checked by muscle response testing. The sublingual test is limited to testing for food items.

Cytotoxic testing is a form of blood test that was developed a few years ago. Many nutritionally oriented practitioners use this test. In this method, an extract of the allergic substance is mixed with a sample of the person's blood, which is then observed under the microscope for changes in white cells. Since foods and other allergic substances do not normally get into the blood in this manner, cytotoxic testing does not give reliable results.

Another very recent blood serum test for allergies is called the "ELIZA" (enzyme linked immuno-zorbent assay) test. In this test, blood serum is tested for various immunoglobulin and their concentrations. The patient has to get exposed to certain foods in a certain amount of time for this test to show some positive results. If the patient has never been exposed to certain foods, this may not show satisfactory results.

The elimination diet, which was developed by Dr. Albert H. Rowe of Oakland, California, consists of a very limited diet which must be followed for a period long enough to determine whether or not any of the foods included in it are responsible for the allergic symptoms. If a fruit allergy is suspected, for example, all fruits are eliminated from the diet for a period which may vary from several days to several weeks. For patients who have suffered allergic symptoms over a period of several years, it is sometimes necessary to abstain from the offending foods for several weeks before the symptoms subside. Therefore, the importance of adhering strictly to the diet during the diagnostic period is very important. When the patient has been free of symptoms for a certain period, other foods are added, one at a time, until a normal diet is attained and the offending foods are discovered.

Another simple way of determining food allergy is by pulse testing. It has been observed that if one eats something to which one is allergic, the pulse rate speeds up. Another way to test for food allergy is by "rotation diet," in which a different group of foods is eaten every day for a week. In this way, seven different groups of foods are eaten in a week, each day something new. Again, the rotation starts from the following Monday. This way one can trace reactions to any group which can then be eliminated. All these diets work most of the time for less reactive people. Someone who is highly allergic to a certain food item, even if he has not touched it for years, can get very sick if he eats that particular food.

There are other allergy treatment methods in practice. Homeopaths believe that if an allergen is introduced to the patient, in minute concentrations at various times, one might build up enough antibodies toward that particular antigen. Eventually, the patient may not get violent reactions to that particular substance. The idea of urine shots works similarly. A patient is asked to eat a particular item, broccoli for example, at different intervals in a day. The urine of that person is collected after a few hours and injected into the body. When a person eats a certain substance the body creates antibodies for that substance and it is excreted in the urine. Then the same urine is injected into the person and his own antibodies are introduced into the body as an injectant. This supposedly builds up more antibodies and eventually the allergic person may not react violently toward the allergen.

All of the above methods work on a certain percentage of people. People who had taken all of these treatments were still found to be allergic to those things when they were tested again by muscle response testing and they had to be treated again by Nambudripad's Allergy Elimination Techniques to make them non-reactive to those allergens.

A 9-year-old girl was known to be allergic to peanuts since her early youth. She was careful not to touch or eat them. One day, at a friend's party, she happened to take a bite of marshmallow puffs in which the hostess had added peanut butter for taste. After the first bite, she got a severe reaction. She could not breathe, her bronchioles tightened. Her mother carried Ventolin spray in her purse all the time for emergency needs, since the child was known to be asthmatic. This time the spray did not help her. Before medical help arrived, she had slipped into a coma just a few minutes after eating the peanut butter marshmallow puff. Just one bite, and she was into a life and death struggle! This shows that elimination and rotation diets do not work for highly allergic patients. Severely allergic patients can suffer from life threatening situations by eating only a bite of an allergen once in their life time.

This girl was in a coma for three months. She had tried all the Western medical treatments, with no positive results. Her desperate parents tried acupuncture on her. Within ten days she awoke from her coma. She was blind, her speech was slurred and her body was flaccid. She could not move or sit on her own. She received Nambudripad's Allergy Elimination Techniques treatment for peanuts and various other allergens for three to four months. At the end of this time she started walking on her own, her speech became clearer, eye sight started improving and returned to normal 13 months after completion of treatment.

A 37-year-old male returned from Mexico after a two week vacation. He woke up at 6 a.m. and rushed to the tennis court for his usual game. While he was warming up, he felt a muscle cramp, first on his right knee, then it started moving upward toward the right thigh, hip joint, then to the lower back. He tumbled down on the court, unable to stand up due to the muscle spasm, and was carried to the nearest medical clinic where he received some muscle relaxant analgesics and therapy. He was sent home with all the medications. The medications helped him for a few minutes, but then muscle spasms returned with severe intensity. His sister, who had previously been treated by Nambudripad's Allergy Elimination Techniques, brought him to our clinic.

From his history it was revealed that he had eaten abalone shellfish three days in a row before he left Mexico. This was the first time he had ever eaten abalone. His pain, muscle spasms and discomfort were relieved completely in fewer than four to five minutes after treatment by Nambudripad's Allergy Elimination Techniques for abalone.

A 6-year-old boy had a low grade fever about 100 to 101 degrees throughout the day for three to four weeks. During this time his parents tried many different treatments, including antibiotics, but nothing gave him relief from his fever. Finally, his mother was able to trace back to the incident that happened four weeks ago, when he drank a glass of eggnog and vomited almost all of it just a few minutes after he drank it. His mother remembered that was also the beginning of his fever. One of the ingredients of the eggnog was nutmeg. He was highly allergic to nutmeg on muscle response testing. After treatment for nutmeg with Nambudripad's Allergy Elimination Techniques, his four week old fever broke and became normal in a couple of hours.

Another 4-year-old girl started vomiting and ran a fever of 103 degrees. Her parents took her to the family doctor and got antibiotics. After three days of oral medication, she did not get better. Her vomiting and fever continued. Finally, she was brought to our clinic. In our clinic it was discovered that she was given cactus pickle by her sitter. She was highly allergic to cactus. After treatment for cactus, she stopped vomiting and her temperature became normal within a few minutes.

A 3 year-old-girl was at a friend's birthday party. After the party all the guests were about to depart. At that time her mother noticed that she could not walk and was crawling on the floor. Her mother thought that she was tired and sleepy due to running and playing the entire evening. She fell asleep in the car. Her parents carried her to the house and to her bed. The next morning, when she refused to wake up, her parents got worried and called the paramedics. The child was still breathing but unresponsive. She was taken to the hospital where she was in a coma. After 72 hours, she woke up to find her lower limbs paralyzed below the waist. She was kept in the hospital nine days, until her general condition stabilized, and was sent home with instructions to follow up with physical therapy for the paralyzed lower limb.

When she was out of the hospital, her parents who were already familiar with Nambudripad's Allergy Elimination Technique, brought her straight to our clinic where it was found that she had eaten a large piece of pineapple cake with chunks of pineapple in it. It was the first time she had ever eaten pineapple. She was found to be allergic to pineapple. She had several treatment sessions by Nambudripad's Allergy Elimination Techniques for pineapple and upon finishing the treatments she started walking on her own. She did not go back for physical therapy. Her temporary paralysis was due to her allergy to pineapple.

An 11-year-old girl got a sore throat and got very sick. Her pediatrician took a throat swab and found that she had strep throat. She took antibiotics for seven days. Instead of getting better, her sore throat got worse. Then she was brought to our clinic. Through a kinesiological examination, we were able to trace the allergen cause of her strep-like symptoms. She had eaten a particular candy bar nine days ago that was the cause of her sore throat. When she was treated for the particular candy bar, her strep-like symptoms cleared in minutes.

A girl 12-years-old suffered from an abdominal cramps every time she ate cauliflower. When she was treated for allergy to cauliflower by NAET, she got rid of her cramps.

A 13 year-old-girl, who had canker sores, was allergic to milk and milk products. She got rid of her canker sores after she was treated for milk products.

A woman 28, who had yeast infections whenever she had an orange, found she was allergic to the vitamin C in the orange.

Another patient, who had complained of shoulder and neck pain most all her life, was allergic to green chili pepper, which was one of her favorite items in salads.

These are a few examples of common problems we see around us every day and are actual case histories from the author's practice.

CHAPTER FOUR

THE LIVING MAZE

The study of the human nervous system is a complicated subject, however, once learned it is one of the most fascinating areas in medicine. The nervous system is a puzzle, a maze that remains largely unsolved because so many of its aspects are not completely understood. It is known, however, that it controls every function of every system in the body. Some basic knowledge about the human nervous system will help the serious reader to understand the relationship between the human body and allergies. More importantly, it opens the door of knowledge to the concepts that lead to treatment of allergies. It allows the reader to make readjustments to the nervous system, rather than depend upon a lifetime of allergy shots, antihistamines, and extensive, expensive types of various allergy treatments.

The nervous system is without doubt, the most complex, widely investigated, and least understood bodily system known to man. Its structures and activities are inseparably interwoven with every aspect of our lives, physical, cultural and intellectual. Accordingly, investigators of many different disciplines, with a variety of methodologies, motivations, and persuasions, converge in its study. Depending on the context, there are also many more or less appropriate ways of embarking upon a study of the nervous system. For example, the approach could be from the developmental point of view or from a variety of other philosophies including, but not limited, to phylogenetic, physiochemical, energetic, structural (gross or cellular), cybernetic, or even behavioral.

For purposes of understanding the relationship between the human body and the nervous system, it is essential that we look at some of the structures and functions of the nervous system that are directly or indirectly involved in the adaptational process. In this section, we will not be concerned with the gross structural aspects of the human nervous system, such as the location of nerve ganglions, trunks, cells, endings, etc., rather the reader is urged to refer to appropriate sections in Gray's or other anatomy texts for such information. In this section, we will try to enlighten you on the chemical and electrical energy aspects only.

GATHERING AND PROCESSING INFORMATION

The human nervous system consists of three parts. The central nervous system, peripheral nervous system, and the autonomic or automatic nervous system. The central nervous system consists of the brain and the spinal cord. The peripheral nervous system consists of all of the nerves that leave the spinal cord and go to muscles and various parts of the body. This includes the motor and sensory nerves that are responsible for muscle movements of the body and also carry the sensations of heat, cold and touch from various parts of the body to the spinal cord. The autonomic nervous system consists of the sympathetic and parasympathetic nervous systems, composed of the nerves regulating the functions of various vital smooth muscles and vital organs such as the heart, lungs, glands, stomach, bladder, colon, etc.

One of the primary functions of the human nervous system is gathering and processing information. Even as one reads this page, conscious gathering and processing of information is taking place. In terms of homeostasis (maintaining a balance with the organism), those who can read this page and find it challenging, or hopefully interesting, will continue to read it or put it aside to read later. Similarly, the person who cannot read will make a conscious decision about it, or perhaps seek a translator to read it, or simply to put it down as a useless exercise. No matter which response is chosen, it is one of consciousness.

In addition to these simple responses to reading this page, the transaction is transmitted along millions of nerve cells or electrical corridors to areas in the brain, where the memory is stored, from which it may be recalled either on command or at the whim of the subconscious mind. For the reader, both conscious recall of the experiences and effects of the subconscious are possible, as a result of contact with this printed page. It is inescapable as we are constantly in process of "becoming" in response to our life experiences.

Just as the total human being senses the stimuli presented by the environment and responds accordingly in a conscious manner, millions of minor adjustments are being made automatically every day with out our conscious decision making. For instance, when we are hot we consciously move ourselves from the sun or turn on the air condition. But unconsciously the body is already making several hundred minor adjustments that trigger changes in the blood flow and the heart rate, expand or contract the blood vessel near the skin surfaces, activate the lymph glands, turn on the sweat glands, and so on. These actions of the autonomic nervous system are reprogrammed into the very cells of the body that respond to conscious activity.

The autonomic responses are reprogrammed to respond appropriately to the changing environment. Sometime, already designed pre-programs produce a similar responses to a large group of stimuli. Consider the human body's reaction to fear.

When we sense a potentially dangerous situation, the autonomic nervous system prepares for a fight or flight reaction. Both are appropriate responses to danger. Again, seconds pass while physical adjustments are snapped into place. Such adjustments include we begin to sweat, our hands become clammy, and beads of perspiration run down from underarms or collects on our foreheads. In addition, the biochemical reaction reduces the blood flow to the head, limiting our thinking and reducing our ability to hear and increases the blood flow to the heart, lungs, and motor muscle tissue. Again, these are all appropriate responses for the body to make in the presence of immediate danger.

The body often is not able to differentiate between physical and physiological or emotional danger. Consequently, we respond involuntarily to a potential mugging in much the same way as we do a job interview, or to a confrontation with an angry dog as we do to a public speaking assignment. In essence, the brain betrays us, because it has developed patterns of responses that are inappropriate to the situation at hand. This is not just an idle philosophical discussion of consciousness, but a foundational premise, upon which an understanding of allergies, the muscle response testing to detect allergies, and the Nambudripad's Allergy Elimination Techniques to eliminate allergies is based upon. The reader may want to read this again.

We have talked about the conscious and the unconscious functioning of the central nervous system, but it is extremely important to recognize the body's attempts to maintain a homeostatic state (balance within the organism). The total balance takes place in various steps, utilizing assistance from a number of functional units. These functional units are large bodies of tissues consisting of collected microscopic cells, each having a specialized job in the body. These special tissues provide assistance in creating homeostasis, at the lowest levels, within the individuals cells themselves.

The process through which this occurs is very complex, requiring considerable understanding of the biochemical and bioelectrical properties of the cells. Simplified, it can be said that all cells are surrounded by a plasma membrane similar to a microscopic plastic bag. The walls of this membrane are thick enough to maintain the cell shape and size and to contain the intracellular materials. It is also strong enough to protect the cells from invasion of the intracellular materials that surrounds each and every cell.

At the same time, it is thin enough and permeable enough to allow free flow of nutrients. The materials inside the cells are quite different from materials outside the cells, particularly in relationship to the ionic or magnetic properties of the atoms that make up these fluids. Because of the differences in ionic composition, it follows that there are differences in their electrical properties. These differences in the electrical energies can be measured in laboratory experiments on various kinds of tissues. But more important to this discussion, millions of similar measurements are made each minute as each individual cell senses the electrical charges and responds according to its specific function in the organism.

As a stimulus is applied at some point on the organism, it sets up a sequence of events that eventually is transmitted to the surfaces of the excitable cells redistributing the ions across the surface. This becomes a transient, reversible wave of change which presumably changes the permeability of cell membranes, allowing a transfer of fluids to take place and changing the cell shape, size or function for a time until it returns to its original or homeostatic state.

While on unicellular life forms, and on some primitive multi-cellular life forms, individual cells are capable of reacting to stimuli; in the majority of complex life forms, in the processing nervous system a division of labor occurs between the excitable cells which make up the system. Thus, in the human body, we have highly specialized receptor cells whose total function is to receive stimuli. These receptor cells function in concert with neurons (nerve cells) for the integration and conduction of information, while effector cells (the contractile and glandular cells) function in the operation of responses to action.

Neurons or nerve cells are stepping stones in the neural pathways. They interact through the use of axons, which carry impulses to neurons; and dendrites, which carry impulses away from the cell body. The ends of various dendrites and axons do not touch to create a wire link; rather, they are interlaced without touching. The space between the ends of the thread-like axons and dendrites are called synapses. The electrical impulses, or energy impulses, jump these spaces in their journey to the brain and back.

Enzymes, a kind of mediator-like cholinesterase, are present on the surface of the neurons and complete the circuits. These enzymes or mediators, are known as neurotransmitters and are extremely important in making intercommunication possible among the cells, neurons, tissues, organs, and different body parts. These neurotransmitters vary among neurons, depending upon the specificity of tissue. Although very different in chemical composition, these enzymes share a common origin. They are produced by the neurons and released into the synapses, when the nerve impulse arrives, which sets off the response in the next cell. Much interest has been shown in these enzymes lately, particularly since they may hold the key to a natural means of controlling pain, addiction to chemicals, aging, disease, the healing mechanism and controlling and eliminating allergies.

The actions and neurological functions of these enzymes in our bodies are still not known completely. Researchers at various institutions and in various fields are trying to understand them. In a few cases, their effects are beginning to be better understood. This is primarily because of the wide distribution throughout the body of such enzymes. These enzymes include mono amino acids known as noradrenalin, serotonin and histamines, all of which have an excitatory effect on the body's nervous system, and dopamine, which has an inhibitory effect.

The ability of the central nervous system to react almost instantaneously to a stimulus; even though it may be only the sensation of heat, cold, smell, etc., on the most remote part of the extremities, is probably the result of the common origin of all parts of the nervous system. The body is made up of trillions of individually well equipped cells. Each cell has the memory to reproduce any number of chemicals and functions in the body. When the cell duplicates, the duplicated cell takes over all the memory of the mother cell. This memory, or duplicating effect, is called deoxyribonucleic acid or DNA. DNA controls the functions of the body through various sensory receptors installed in each cell surface. This DNA, and the other characteristics of the individual cells, were duplicated and carried over from the beginning of the unicellular life. Since the body formed from a single cell, identical or duplication of the memory in each cell is made possible.

The embryonic ectoderm gives rise to all of the nervous system, including the central nervous system, peripheral nervous system, and autonomic nervous system, sensory and touch receptors, etc. It is this origin that accounts for the body's ability to function as a unit, each part corresponding to another, through the central nervous system, using the sensory receptors. When one of the sensory receptors senses something in the functional unit that is within the body, the message is passed on to the central nervous system. From there, the message goes to each and every cell of the body through the centrifugal or efferent nerve fibers. The whole body, including trillions of neurons and cells is then alerted to accept or reject the stimulus.

If the stimulus or message reaches the brain; providing it is not short-circuited by nerve damage, blockage, or missed chemical response due to some defect in the neurotransmitters, the brain accepts the message. Then it formulates and transmits a response to all other receptors in the body. In turn, the receptors may receive the message as harmful or harmless. If the receptors receive the message as harmful, those particular receptors repel it and confirm their findings to the brain. If more stimuli with negative reactions reach the brain, the brain accepts the rejection message from the majority of receptors. Since the brain's responses are impartial, the receptors corresponding to the area of the stimuli will react accordingly and set in motion evasive actions. In the worst case scenario, where the body cannot effectively avoid or reject the stimulus, it will set up a reaction in an effort to cleanse the body of the stimulus.

For the most part, the nervous system producing negative responses to a stimulus; especially to an allergic stimulus, is the automatic nervous system. It consists of two parts, the parasympathetic and the sympathetic, as we discussed earlier. Physiologically, parasympathetic reactions are localized. They result in slowing of the heart rate and increased glandular and peristaltic action of the gut and other hollow organs. Sympathetic activities, on the other hand, are exhibited as mass responses to stimuli and include constriction of the blood vessels under the skin, which increases the blood flow to the heart, lungs, muscles, and brain, accelerates the heart rate, increases blood pressure, and decreases peristalsis (kneading action of the gut), etc.

Activities of the sympathetic system prepare the body for increased activities. Biochemically, the action of the sympathetic system is characterized by the formation of noradrenalin and adrenalin, along with some other basic enzymes, to prepare the body for reaction.

The sympathetic nerves exit from the thoracic region of the spinal column. That is why chiropractors, who specialize in the study of the spinal column, can perform miraculous cures in certain patients without the use of any medications. Either side of the spinal column, half an inch to one inch away from the spine, is a group of important acupuncture points. They are directly related to the vital organs and organ functions. When an acupuncturist stimulates these points with the acupuncture needle, the similar miraculous results happen in the sick people.

Chiropractors and acupuncturists are stimulating the sympathetic nerve activity, thus removing the nerve energy blockages to reinstate the nerve energy circulation in the body. These two groups of medical practitioners from East and West have learned to manipulate the sympathetic nerves to the patient's advantage and promote the healing power within the body itself, without the introduction of foreign chemicals.

Beyond this point, the nervous system becomes a matter of complicated medical study. It is sufficient to say, however, from this understanding of the mechanics of the nervous system that a very minor stimulus at any receptor nerve cell location on the body will set in motion the manufacturing process of hundreds of different kinds of chemicals that assist the nerves in producing the appropriate responses to the stimulus.

CHAPTER FIVE

KINESIOLOGY AND ACUPUNCTURE

The word "kinesiology" actually means the science of movement and was first proposed by Dr. George Goodhart, a Detroit doctor of chiropractic medicine in 1964. As a function of his practice, Dr. Goodheart learned a great deal about a patient's condition using techniques which isolated the movements of various muscles. The isolation techniques, a chiropractic procedure, make it possible to test the strength of an individual muscle or muscle group without the help of other muscles. Dr. Goodheart, with the help of Dr. Hetrick and others, came to the conclusion, after many experiments, that structural imbalance leads to disorganization of the entire body. The disorganization results in specific disorders of the glands, organs, and central nervous system, similar to what pioneer Chinese doctors had observed.

Kinesiology holds that when the body is disorganized, the structural balance or electrical forces are not functioning in a normal way. When this happens, the central nervous system sends out a signal that is directed at each and every cell of the body, because each cell in the body is directly connected with the brain via a network of nerves. These sensory and motor nerve cells reach every cell of the body and are capable of conducting messages back and forth with the brain at all times and are under the direct command of the brain. The electrical energy, or the life force, flows through these nerve cells, which makes energy channels. This energy is called different names by different people. In Chinese it is called "chi", in Sanskrit and Hindustani it is "prana," in English it is called "life force" or "vital energy." Using a more simple term, we call it energy.

According to the Chinese, free flow of energy is necessary for the normal functioning of the body. When the energy gets blocked, or when the free flow gets obstructed, one becomes ill. The messages from the brain or to the brain also pass through this energy channel. The energy travels from cell to cell in split milliseconds. Along with the energy, the messages are also communicated.

Pioneer Chinese doctors and philosophers had studied these energy pathways, and networks of the energy system of the human body, many years ago by observing living people and their normal and abnormal body functions. The Chinese had learned to manipulate these energy pathways or meridians to the body's advantage. In olden days, about 4,000 years ago, there was no scientific equipment available to feel or sense the presence of the energy flow and its pathways. Now, it is possible to study and trace the energy flows and pathways by using Kirlian photography and radioactive tracer isotopes. Having confirmed the existence of energy pathways in the human body, the Chinese doctors hypothesized and established the existence of these pathways long ago.

According to Chinese medical theory, any obstruction in the energy flow in the pathways can cause imbalance in the body. Any imbalance can cause illness. To remove the imbalance, the cause has to be removed. If energy blockage is the cause of the imbalance, when the blockage is removed the balance will be reinstated. When the body is in perfect balance, it can not experience any illness. When acupuncture needles are placed at various points in the acupuncture meridians, energy blockage is removed temporarily, and the state of balance is achieved. That is how acupuncture treats various ailments.

According to Chinese medical theory, free-flowing chi through the meridians is necessary to keep the body in perfect balance. In the United States in the 19th century, Daniel David Palmer, founder of chiropractic medicine said, "Too much or too little energy is sickness." His theory corresponded with the ancient

Chinese theory of "free flow of energy," even though Palmer probably had no idea about Chinese medicine or its existence.

In this country, chiropractic medicine developed under Palmer. The chiropractors learned about the "too much energy or too little energy," and how to bring the body to a balanced state by manipulating the spinal segments and the spinal nerve roots and keeping them in perfect alignment. In the East, acupuncture took its roots based on the ancient Chinese theory, and acupuncturists tried to bring the body into perfect balance by manipulating the energy pathways at various acupuncture points by inserting acupuncture needles to remove blockages in the meridians and thus reinstate the " free flow of chi" along the energy pathways. East and West, without being aware of each other's findings, worked in a similar manner toward the same purpose, i.e., to balance the energy and to free sick people from their misery.

Both groups realized that the cause of imbalance is energy disturbance, which can be due to overflow or underflow. When the flow is reinstated, the balance is also restored. How can we remove the cause of blockage? If we can eliminate the primary cause for the blockage, there is no need for the body to go into an unbalanced state. Then, the body does not have to experience sickness. The Chinese knew that the causes of blockages are many. The main ones being physical, physiological, as well as psychological disturbances. They tried to protect patients from these problems, but it was not easy to avoid the causes, so they concentrated mainly on removing the blockages.

When there is an energy blockage in the pathway, there will be stagnation on one side and poor flow on the other. When there is stagnation, there will be back flow, which then will become overflow through various connecting meridians. All the meridians or energy pathways are associated with various major vital organs. The backflow and overflow will affect these organs directly or indirectly. The stagnation of energy can be seen or felt as localized aches, pains, or discomfort; backflow or overflow can be seen as vital organ malfunctions or "excess" syndromes. Underflow, on the other side of the blockage, also affects another group of meridians and their related organs. The hypo-functions of those organs, or deficiency syndromes of those organs, can be felt as a result.

A trained acupuncturist can determine and differentiate between the overflow and underflow of chi and its affected meridians and organs. When treatment is administered to strengthen the underflowing or hypofunctioning organ, and to drain the overflowing meridians and the organs, balance is achieved faster. This is the practice of acupuncture. Muscle response testing and Nambudripad's Allergy Elimination Techniques are built on acupuncture theory, but they have taken it one step further. This was probably one of the missing links the various professionals were searching for over the years and could not find. Muscle response testing and Nambudripad's Elimination Techniques will be discussed in later chapters.

To recap, energy blockage happens due to some disturbance in the energy system. Earth has its own magnetic energy which is also called gravity. All objects in this universe have their own energy fields. Every object, living or non living, has an electromagnetic field around it. Objects on earth have an attraction or repulsion among themselves. In reality, there should not be any repulsion between objects, because they are all part of the universe and they are meant to be together in unison. Man, being a part of the universe, should not have any repulsion toward any objects around him, but due to genetic mutation and changes in the environment, the energy field of man has changed. This altered state makes him incompatible with various objects around him. When any of these substances get close to him, energy disturbance takes place. When there is an energy disturbance in the energy pathways, energy blockage results. This causes the body to go into an unbalanced state and eventually the whole body, including meridians, vital organs and associated muscle groups, all become involved and disorganized.

The central nervous system instantly responds to the presence of the substance that caused the blockage of an energy pathway and perceives that substance to be toxic and harmful to the body. The brain acts and works like the most efficient of computers. Any kinetic changes or movements in the cells are recorded in the brain's computer instantly. In the future, whenever the body comes in contact with that particular object, the brain will perceive it to be toxic and harmful and will call its defensive forces into action. One of the brain's primary functions is to take care of the body's welfare, so whenever the brain senses an item to be harmful to the body, it tries to eliminate it to protect the body.

Most of the time the responses are hidden, masked by hundreds of simultaneous responses taking place every instance. When isolated, both in terms of contact with the toxin and the muscles and organs affected, a particular response to the toxic substance can be observable and definable. The super-computer, the brain, registers each and every movement of each cell of the body every time. When the presence of an unsuitable item causes an energy disturbance in the energy pathway, the flow of energy is blocked, the body goes into imbalance, and the normal bodily functions do not proceed as they should. These changes and disturbances are directly sensed and recorded by the brain through its abundant sensory nerve fibers present at various parts of the body. The normal flow of energy regulates and controls all bodily functions, including the functions of the immune systems in the body. When there is an energy disturbance, all the bodily functions are alerted, and the brain records the event as the cause of the disturbance in its memory.

For example, when one is exposed to a substance such as strawberries and the brain happens to perceive strawberries as a cause of an energy disturbance, this knowledge is recorded in the brain's computer instantly. The next time the body gets near a strawberry, the brain will sense the danger instantly and summon its defense forces to work to help get rid of the substance that cause the energy disturbance and thus an imbalance and sickness in the body. Most people who are allergic to strawberries react violently upon eating the berries. Sneezing and a runny nose represent an effort on the part of these organs to throw off some irritant already inside the body. When giant hives occur, watery fluid is present in the tissue, and severe vomiting and diarrhea occur, this may be due to the action of various defense forces working in the body to get rid of the toxins that have entered it.

As long as energy flows freely through the energy pathways, one cannot get sick, but any physical, physiological and psychological trauma can cause disturbance in the flow of energy along the meridians. The presence of any allergic substances like food items, fabrics, animals or materials can be included in the category of items that can cause physical disturbances causing energy blockage. After effects of ingesting allergic foods, alcohol, drugs, etc., may be included in the category of the causes of physiological disturbances. For example, too much sodium chloride consumption can cause fluid retention in the body. Fluid retention can cause swelling of the tissues; swelling of the tissues can irritate the nerves and cause pain and discomfort in the body. This will, in turn, disturb the physiological function of other organs and cause imbalance in the whole body.

The third category of items that produce imbalance is psychological or emotional disturbances. Extreme joy, anger, shocking or sad news, sudden loss of loved ones, huge financial losses; natural disturbances such as fire, earthquakes, etc., can cause energy disturbances and blockages and hence imbalances in the meridians, organs, and associated muscle groups. If one uses or eats any allergenic item while the body is in such unbalanced state, the body experiences the pangs of allergic reaction in many forms and degrees.

If the body did not experience a major trauma, the allergies would probably have remained hidden or less reactive. When the body is in balance, most of the allergies do not exhibit their usual reactions. That is why most of the allergic manifestations follow a major trauma or a major event in one's life, such as an automobile or other accident, major illnesses, loss of a loved one, or financial or job loss, etc.

When one experiences a major trauma, the body uses all of its defense forces to overcome the trauma. In trying to save the body from the trauma, it exhausts its entire reservoir of strength. At this time, if the allergy attacks the body, the body is unable to defend itself and becomes a convenient victim of an allergic attack. During this process, the immune system becomes exhausted, the blockages enlarge, the stagnation and backflow or overflow or underflow become exaggerated in the body, energy blockages start affecting the tissues and organs. Temporary changes turn into permanent changes in various organs, the body is overcome by various diseases and symptoms like migraine headaches, asthma, emphysema, arthritis, lung disorders, tumors, carcinomas, epstein-barr viruses, tuberculosis, and other immune deficiency disorders. From this explanation, one can see that sickness starts with simple imbalances in the body due to blockages in the energy flow.

Acupuncture, on certain points, will help to drain the blockages out of the body by creating an exit via the insertion of the needle. Adverse energy, from the allergen that causes blockages in the human body meridians, will turn into heat. This heat, under pressure, causes tension. When the needle is inserted, the heat, under pressure, will get a chance to exit because metal needles have the ability to transfer heat from inside to outside or from highly heated areas to low heated areas.

Heat from inside the body will not exit through skin, because under the skin we have the best insulation one can ever find. That is why a needle is needed to draw out the built up heat from the inside layers. Expulsion of heat can be seen with the naked eye around the inserted acupuncture needle as redness, red welts, or a red pimple, immediately after the needle insertion. The larger the red areas the more heat is accumulated in the body, and the case is said to be in an excess condition.

Kinesiology and acupuncture have so much in common, because, the development of the former was based on acupuncture theory. Perhaps the ancient Chinese doctors knew about kinesiology muscle testing, although there is no written trace or proof of such knowledge. Most of the pioneer Chinese doctors did not share all their knowledge with their peers or students for fear of losing their power and position. Possibly this very important knowledge has been buried and disappeared with the passing years. In any case, Chinese scientists' knowledge of the structure of the nervous system and circulatory system of the blood is apparent in their placement of acupuncture points.

Herbs also will do the same healing. Electromagnetic forces of special herbs actually have the quality to enter the selective meridians and the strong electrical forces of these herbs can push energy blockages out of the body and restore the energy balances. The well trained herbologist can bring the same result as acupuncture. Acupuncture and herbs together can produce excellent results also. If the herbologist is not well trained, he can cause more damages to the meridians, should he fail to diagnose or find the exact blocked meridian and give the herbs to clear the wrong meridians.

Ignorance is the worst enemy of progress. Western medical doctors depend on the latest scientific tools and medicines. Most Western doctors are not encouraged to look at the body and study its own power of natural healing. If given a chance, appropriate stimulation, to the body and brain can produce substances within the body including endorphins, enkaphalins, and immune mediators to heal many problems. The brain can heal infections, allergies, tuberculosis immune deficiency diseases, etc. This has been demonstrated repeatedly and proven in many cases treated by Nambudripad's techniques. It is necessary to raise the level of the immune system, then the full power of the brain and the body to heal itself comes forward. Your body can form antibodies to clear these unsolved health problems when the immune system is functioning optimally and the body is in optimum balance. If all medical professionals from different fields would get together and learn each others different techniques and practices together, all the holistic and Oriental knowledge and Western medical knowledge would compliment one another and millions of suffering people all over the world would see some light at end of the tunnel.

In any case, this NEW technique is a blessing mainly to the multitudes of sufferers from allergies whom it helps. Kinesiology and acupuncture both help sick people immensely by removing energy blockages from energy pathways by various kinesiological techniques and acupuncture needles. They also help well people maintain their health by preventing the causes of energy blockages. Both these disciplines also tried to maintain good health by promoting good nutrition, good living habits, good mental attitudes and exercise.

CHAPTER SIX

MUSCLE RESPONSE TESTING FOR ALLERGIES

Muscle response testing is one of the tools used by kinesiologists to test the kinetic imbalances in the body. The same muscle response test can also be used to detect various allergens that cause imbalances in the body.

As we saw earlier, when the allergens' incompatible electromagnetic energy comes close to one's energy field, repulsion takes place. Without recognizing this repulsive action, we go near allergens whether they be foods, drinks, chemicals or animals and tangle with their energies. This causes energy blockages in the meridians. The blockage causes imbalances and disorganization in the body. The blockage also causes stagnation and illness. This disorganization in the body involves the vital organs and their associated muscle groups.

In response, to prevent the allergen from entering into deeper levels, after causing the internal energy blockages, the message from the brain reaches each and every cell of the body to reject the presence of the allergen. This will appear as repulsion, and the person's weakness can show up as tiredness, aches and pains or many other unpleasant symptoms.

Our bodies have an amazing way of telling us when we are in trouble. As a matter of practice, we have to be hurting severely before we look for help. If we went for help at the earliest hint of need, we would not have to suffer the pain and agony. This applies to allergies too. If we find our allergies before we are exposed to them, we will not have to suffer the consequences. If we understand our bodies, brain and their clues, we can avoid the causes that contribute to the energy blockages and imbalances in the body.

A nine year old girl was being treated for asthma by Nambudripad's Allergy Elimination Techniques. She was treated for various items, and she was able to eat them without getting an asthmatic attack. One day her parents took her to a Chinese restaurant. When the food was brought to the table, she immediately whispered to her mother that she thought she was allergic to some of the food items on the plate and that she might become ill if she ate the food. The girl's mother ignored her and forced her to eat the food saying that she had been treated for it. Before she finished eating, she had an asthmatic attack. The confused mother brought a sample to the office of everything the child ate. She was found to be allergic to the mixed vegetables which had a great deal of corn starch. The nine year old was smart enough to recognize the allergen before she ate it. She said, as soon as the food was placed in front of her, her throat started itching and this gave her a clue that she might be allergic to something on the plate.

When some people are near allergens or adversely charged substances they get various clues from the brain, such as itchy throat or eyes, sneezing attacks, coughing spells, unexpected pain anywhere in the body, yawning, sudden tiredness, etc. These weaknesses of the body, in the presence of an allergen, can be demonstrated by testing a strong indicator muscle in the absence and presence of an allergen. The muscle will be strong without any allergens and will go weak in the presence of an allergen. This response of the muscle can be used to our advantage to demonstrate the presence of an allergen near us.

SEE ILLUSTRATIONS OF MUSCLE RESPONSE TESTING ON THE FOLLOWING PAGES.

MUSCLE RESPONSE TESTING

Muscle response testing can be done in two ways. First, as the standard muscle response test, and second as the oval ring test or 'O' ring test in which the individual tests himself.

To perform standard muscle response testing two people are required. The person who performs the test is called the tester, and the person on whom the test is performed is called the subject. The subject can be tested lying down, standing or sitting positions. The lying down position is more convenient for the tester and the subject and gives more accurate results.

Step 1: The subject lies on a firm surface face, with one hand raised 90 degrees to his body and his thumb facing toward his big toe, or palm facing outward.

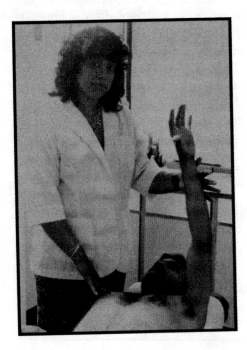

Step 2:   The tester stands on the subject's side opposite the raised arm and gently rests one hand on the shoulder of the resting for balance.

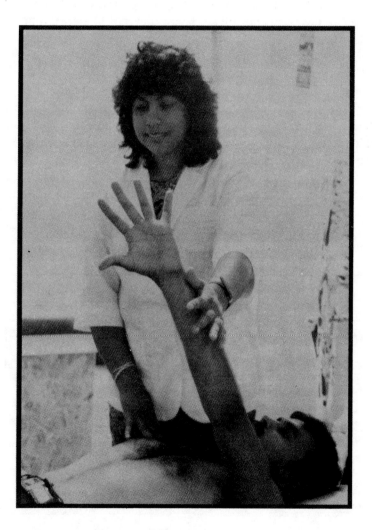

Step 3: The tester, using his free arm, tries to push down on the raised arm of the subject toward the subject's toe. The subject resists the push of the tester on his arm (the indicator muscle). The indicator muscle remains strong if the subject is well-balanced at the time of testing. It is essential to test a strong indicator muscle to get accurate results. If the muscle or raised arm is weak and gives away on pressure, the subject is probably not balanced, or the tester may not be performing the test properly.

For example, the tester might be trying to overpower the subject. There is no need to overpower the subject, and the subject shouldn't need to gather up strength from other muscles in the body to resist the tester with all his might. The tester needs to apply only about five to ten pounds of pressure on the muscle for about three to five seconds. If the muscle shows weakness, the tester will be able to judge the difference with that much pressure. A lot of practice is needed to test and sense the differences properly. There is no need to get discouraged or frustrated if one cannot test properly or effectively the first few times.

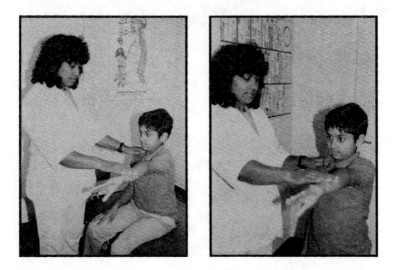

Step 4: If the subject is found to be balanced, and if the indicator muscle remains strong on test, put the suspected allergen into the subject's palm of the resting hand. The sensory receptors on the palmer side, at the tip of the fingers are extremely sensitive to recognize the allergens. These fingertips have specialized sensory receptors and can send messages to and from the brain. These receptors function as eyes for the blind and convey the messages to the brain almost as the seeing man's eyes do. When the subject touches the allergen with the fingertips, the sensory receptors sense the charges of the allergen and gives a message to the brain. If it is an incompatible charge, the strong indicator muscle will go weak. If the charges are compatible to the body, the indicator muscle will remain strong. This way, one can test any number of items to determine the compatible and incompatible charges.

REBALANCING ILLUSTRATION

This procedure is used if the patient is found to be out of balance which is indicated when indicator muscle or raised arm is weak without an allergen. The tester then places his or her fingertips of one hand on the mid-line of the subject, about one and a half inches below the navel (point 1). The other hand is placed on conception (Ren) Vessel 17 (point 2), in the center of the chest on the mid-line, level with the nipple line. He taps these two points with the fingertips about 20 or 30 seconds, then repeats steps 2 and 3. If the indicator muscle tests strong, continue on to step 4. If the indicator muscle tests weak again, repeat this procedure for two to three times more. It is very unlikely that one person will remain weak after repeating this procedure for two to three times.

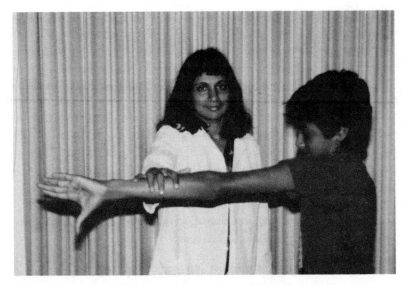

Testing in Standing Position

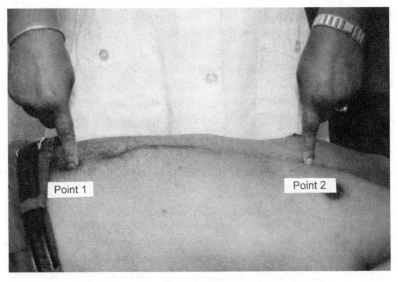

Point 1   Point 2

Picture shows how to balance a patient

Point 1: One and a half inches below the navel, on the mid-line, is called the "sea of energy." This is where the energy of the body is stored in abundance. For some reason, when the body experiences energy blockages, the energy supply is cut short and stored here. If one taps on that energy reservoir point, the energy starts bubbling up and comes out of hiding.

Point 2: Is called "dominating energy." This is the point which controls and regulates the qi, or energy circulation, in the body. When the energy rises from the "sea of energy," it goes straight to the "dominating qi" point. From here, the energy is sent to different meridians as needed to help remove the energy blockages by forcing energy circulation from inside out. During this forced energy circulation, the blockages are pushed out of the body, and the body comes to a balanced state, which we sense through the strong indicator muscle.

OVAL RING, OR "O" RING TEST

Some people are able to test themselves as shown below after considerable practice.

Step A: The tester (him or herself) makes an "O" shape by opposing his little finger and thumb on one hand. Then with the other index finger, he or she tries to separate the "O" ring against pressure. If the ring separates easily, one needs to use the balancing techniques as described in step 5 of the muscle response test.

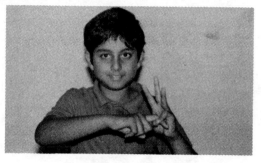

Step B: If the "O" ring remains inseparable and strong, hold the allergen in the other hand, touching it with the finger tips, and perform step 1 again. If the "O" ring separates easily, the person is allergic to the substances he is touching. If the "O" ring remains strong, he is not allergic to the substance.

SURROGATE TESTING

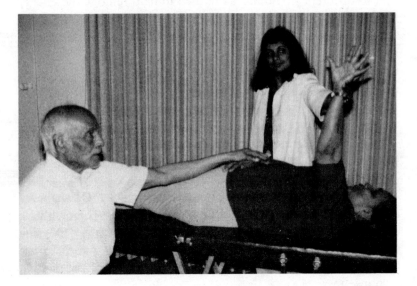

Surrogate Testing Method

This can be used to determine the allergies of a small child, an infant or invalid. Muscle response testing is done through a surrogate. The surrogate lies down and the tester tests the surrogate's raised arm while the subject is touching the surrogate's body. Energy from the subject flows through the surrogate, and the weakness or strength can be seen in the surrogate's body.

This is a very helpful tool to test an old and debilitated person or the very young, who do not have enough muscle strength to perform an allergy test. Muscle response testing is one of the most reliable, most easily performed tests for allergies available. Expensive laboratory work, uncomfortable and painful blood work or skin tests are not necessary to perform muscle response testing. There is no need to wait days and weeks before the results are found. This test can be performed on infants, children, the old and debilitated and strong persons at any time in the privacy of one's own home. If learned properly and practiced correctly, this can save one's life in dangerous situations.

As mentioned earlier, muscle response testing is one of the tools used by kinesiologists all over the world. Practiced in this country since 1964, it was originated by Dr. George Goodheart and his associates. Dr John Thie has tried his best to reach the whole world through the "Touch For Health" foundation in Pasadena, California. For more information, interested readers can write to "Touch For Health" Foundation, where various books are available on the subject.

Any substance can be tested for allergies by muscle response testing. Human beings also can be tested for each other in this manner. The subject lies down, touches the other person he or she wants to get tested. The tester pushes the arm of the subject as in steps 2 and 3. If the subject is allergic to the second person, the indicator muscle goes weak. If the subject is not allergic, the indicator muscle remains strong. Animals, pets, etc., can also be tested this way.

Many infants spit up or vomit milk after they drink it. Some infants get severe colic, crying spells, sleep disorders, constipation, etc. When this happens, pediatricians usually change the milk formula and try others until the infant gets better and does well with one that suits them. If the infants continue to throw up all their food, in extreme cases, surgery is performed to tighten up the cardiac end of the stomach so that whatever the child drinks will hopefully remain in the stomach. In such cases his misery will just be beginning. Allergies build up and problems start one after another. Eventually, the child spends his entire life with repeated surgeries and endless misery.

A 28 year old woman came to our office with complaints of severe migraine headaches. She got a headache once a week or so, which kept her in bed in a dark room with medications, and most of the time with pain shots as well for at least two days. On examination of her history, it was revealed that she had 32 surgeries in her 28 years of life. She had hernia surgery when she was an infant, seven surgeries for gastric ulcers, six on both knees, two on her nose, two on her sinuses, four on her shoulders, one to remove a cyst from her ovaries, two to remove lumps in her ankle, two on the bladder, one on the ear, one on the throat to remove her tonsil. She felt as if there were a big mass on one side of her head whenever she had a migraine on either side of her head. Brain swelling was the cause of this pseudo-mass. Finally she was advised to have brain surgery to prevent the severe debilitating migraine.

Muscle response testing revealed she was highly allergic to every substance around her. She was treated by Nambudripad's Allergy Elimination Techniques for almost a year, at the rate of five treatments a week. Treatments includes testing for almost every item she might come in contact with, the first few treatments concentrating on her regular food items. Then she was treated for her usual clothing items. By the end of three months her migraines were almost gone. If she got one at all, it was with much less intensity and for a much shorter duration. At the end of one year she was almost a normal person who could come out of her shell and live like other normal human beings.

Incidentally, toward the end of the treatment, she met a young man and fell in love for the first time in her life. A year after that they got married and they now lead a normal happy life. This is one of the happy endings to a miserable situation.

There are thousands of people who still suffer like her, running from doctor to doctor, surgery to surgery for problem after problem, exhausting their finances, interest and enthusiasm for life. If we could only teach the medical professionals and the public alike about the importance of allergies and simple tools to locate them, we would probably not have to witness or suffer so many "incurable" health hazards.

Medical professionals and the public alike should be educated to listen and look for various types of allergies when one cannot find the cause of a problem. Unless one is educated to know about something, one does not know what to look for. As we have seen, the theory of energy blockages and diseases comes from Oriental medicine. Oriental medicine also teaches that if given a chance, the body will heal by itself with a little support from herbs or acupuncture in removing blockages.

CHAPTER SEVEN

CAUSES OF DISEASE

As mentioned earlier, imbalances are caused by energy blockages or obstructions of energy circulation along the energy pathways, otherwise known as meridians. The obstruction of energy can be caused by either internal or external factors.

Internal factors arise within the body itself and may be due to dysfunctions of vital organs (i.e., heart attacks, liver failure, lung disorders such as asthma, emphysema; kidney problems, digestive problems, genito-urinary problems, abnormal growths, brain disorders, etc.). It can also be due to emotional disturbances such as excessive reaction of joy, sudden sad news or grief, etc.; nutritional deficiencies or excessive overeating, or eating of unsuitable or uncooked foods etc. The prolonged effect of external factors may also turn into internal factors.

External factors causing energy blockages are, for example, eating unsuitable foods and drinks, environmental materials like pollens, and airborne bacteria, viruses or any other disease-producing agents, fabrics, clothing (wool, cotton, synthetic materials), insect bites, local application of cosmetics, etc.
All of these external factors can turn into internal problems and may cause illness, if not taken care of right away.

Diseases contributed by various allergens can enter the body in many ways. They may enter through the mouth via ingestion, by nose via inhalation, by skin via injection and local application and osmosis. They can also enter the body via ingestion by nerve endings, by conduction or transfer of electromagnetic energy, through fabrics, jewelry, metals, etc. All substances have an electromagnetic charge around them as man has around him. Therefore, nearly all of these substances are capable of affecting the human body in a negative or positive way by transference of the electromagnetic charges alone.

When an unsuitable electrical charge or an allergen; whether it be food, drink, materials, fabrics, animals or another human being, comes near the body, there will be a clash in their fields. There will be a large force of repulsion between the charges. This repulsion creates blockages of the meridians or energy pathways. The sudden blocking of the meridians is one of the quickest defense mechanisms of the brain to stop the allergen from entering deeper into the body and thus prevent imbalances and sickness. This is because one of the prime functions of the brain is to protect the body from any factor that the brain senses as harmful to the body.

Repulsion between charges causes blockages in the meridians. The greater the difference in the charges, the greater the repulsion and the blockage, leading to greater imbalances or disorganization in the body. When severe disorganization takes place in the body, energy does not flow freely in the meridians. When energy does not flow freely in the meridians, stagnation takes place. This follows backflow, overflow and under flow of energy in certain areas of the meridians. When this happens, bodily functions do not proceed properly.

When bodily functions do not take place freely, the body begins to experience health problems, such as aches, pains in the body, sore throat, mildly feverish sensations, chills, painful lymph nodes, muscle pain, weakness, extreme fatigue, headaches in different parts of the head, sleep disturbances, irritability, forgetfulness, confusion, depression, difficulty in thinking or concentrating, phobias, crying spells, suicidal behavior, loneliness even in crowds, sores in the mouth, indigestion, bloating, frequent urination or water retention in the body, burning sensation anywhere in the body, especially on the limbs (hands, feet, palms and soles). These symptoms are experienced immediately after the energy gets blocked with allergens.

If one fails to discover the cause of the blockage, and the blockage continues, the adverse energy eventually takes over the body and causes problems at deeper levels. For example, the aches and pains can turn into chronic arthritis causing degenerative changes in the joints and organs; a sore throat can turn into an infection in the throat, a growth or enlarged tonsils not cured by surgery; painful lymph nodes may turn into puss filled abscesses, breast abscesses into tumors and cancers; muscle weakness may turn into wasting disorders; simple headaches into severe migraines; simple sleep disorders may turn into severe insomnia; neuropsychological complaints like anger, irritability, confusion, depression, etc., might turn the sufferer into a severe psychiatric case and finally lead to a mental institution.

Most practitioners and patients must be familiar with these problems seen at the initial stage of blocked energy flows. Most people identify these symptoms as "chronic fatigue syndrome," a debilitating disease for which no successful treatment has been found by Western medicine.

We treated a 28-year-old computer programmer, who began to feel extreme fatigue, a year after he started working with a well known computer firm. He had a wife and two handsome children. When he started experiencing incompacitating exhaustion, especially toward the end of the day, he started hating to go to work. His output started slowing down; he was diagnosed as having extreme "chronic fatigue syndrome." He reached the point of not even being able to walk without assistance. Finally he had to go on disability insurance. When he was away from work for a while, he started feeling better. When he went back to work, his problems started all over, even though he was given regular physical therapy and supportive treatments.

Finally four years later, when he was seen in our office, it was discovered that he was highly allergic to plastic products and his computer keyboard. He was also allergic to computer radiation.

After he was treated by Nambudripad's Allergy Elimination Techniques for plastics, keyboard, and radiation, he was able to resume his regular work again.

A 30-year-old housewife, who worked as a dressmaker in her spare time, began complaining of severe chronic fatigue syndrome and severe bursitis at the right shoulder joint and pain in the elbow joint. She was listless most of the time, with no energy or enthusiasm to do anything, and felt highly irritated with her two children, one seven and the other nine. She could not do her normal household chores suffering from weakness in her limbs. Her understanding husband employed a part-time house-keeper to help with her chores and to take care of the children. But her complaints got worse and she was getting weaker and weaker. She started getting severe debilitating migraine headaches and became almost completely dependant on pain medications. After a while, even pain medications did not give her any relief.

When she was seen in our office, during one of her interviews, she informed us that she still did some sewing in the afternoon as that was her most enjoyable hobby. That gave us a clue to do more investigation into her mysterious sickness. She also had a bad right shoulder, which was diagnosed as bursitis and calcification in the shoulder. When she was tested she was found to be very allergic to the sewing needle. She was also mildly allergic to the sewing materials. She was also found to be allergic to the needlework frame. The frame was made up of wood, and the needle contained iron. She was found to be very allergic to iron and wood, which were the cause of her unusual sickness. When she was treated for the needle, stainless steel, iron and wood, she began recovering from her debilitating illness. It took a few more months for her to get back to normal.

A 30-year-old nurse had a similar problem. She complained of a severe tenosynovitis (pain in the thumb and metacarpal joint) of both hands, more severe on the right hand, that progressed and radiated into the elbow and shoulder joints. She had nine months of physical therapy and many analgesics but nothing gave her relief. She was referred to our office by her treating physician. When we saw her in our office, she was on disability from her work because of excruciating pain and an inability to perform her nursing duties. She had severe insomnia due to pain and suffered from asthma. She was treated for various allergens in our office with Nambudripad's Allergy Elimination Techniques. Her asthma improved considerably and she slept better at night. Her energy also increased.

After two months of continuous treatment, her original problem of tenosynovitis and bursitis did not get any better. During a reevaluation interview, and on questioning in greater detail, it was discovered that she cooked every day for her husband and three children. While cutting the vegetables and meat, she often used a crude pig-iron knife (black and coarse), which she had brought especially from India because she liked its sharpness. She was asked to bring this knife for testing and she was found to be very allergic to it. She took about seven consecutive treatments with NAET to clear the allergy for that crude iron knife. When the treatment was successfully completed, her aching joints returned to normal. Seven years later, at the time of this writing, she still continues to be symptom-free.

A 33-year-old, who was seen in our office, had the following history. She was married 12 years ago. A week after her marriage, she developed a strange problem. Her left hand went numb and later she began experiencing severe shooting pains in her left arm and joints. She was seen by orthopedic and neuro-logical doctors many times, and her hand was x-rayed a few times. Finally, she said a chiropractor gave her some relief of that pain and discomfort, but it did not last long. She started having more numbness on the same hand and fingers. Then her numbness turned into excruciating pain in the left fingers, left forearm, left elbow and shoulder joints.

Finally, the pain started affecting her spine, mainly in the upper back. She became a regular visitor to the chiropractor's office, sometimes twice a day. She had to use a sling on her left arm to support it. She even started having pain in the right arm. Along with the pain syndrome, she started getting severe bronchitis and regular attacks of pneumonia. When she was seen in our office in 1985, she was in very poor physical condition. She was first treated for various food allergies, which eliminated her chronic upper respiratory infections and bronchitis, but the pain in her left arm remained. Sometimes she said acupuncture helped her.

On one of her usual visits to the office, her painful points were traced by palpation by the doctor to determine where to insert acupuncture needles. To her surprise, the radiation of the pain was traced to the ring finger. Instantly, she was asked to remove her large single stone diamond ring to test for allergies. She was slightly superstitious, but she reluctantly took it off to perform the test. She felt guilty taking off the ring and said she had made a vow never to remove that wedding ring from her finger. She needed her loving and understanding husband's moral support before she removed it.

Now it was this couple's turn to be taken by surprise. The lady was highly allergic to this "diamond ring to be worn forever." Diamond is a stone with a powerful electromagnetic force field. After this discovery, she quit wearing it as an experiment. In two days' time, she stopped hurting in the left arm and upper back. She tried to wear the ring few times, but each time the excruciating pain in the left arm returned. Finally, when she was treated successfully for the diamond, which took

17 consecutive treatments. Then she was able to wear it without pain.

Incidentally, one of the author's childhood memories might interest some diamond lovers. A 36 year old, very successful businessman, decided to buy a large diamond ring for prestige. Indians love jewelry, especially gold and precious stones, and many of them love to show off with the largest stones they can get. Tom found a ring with a large stone, which made him happy. In the store he slipped the ring on his finger and walked toward his car. Before he opened the car door, he had a heart attack, fell on the road and died before any medical help could get to him. Some people gossiped that he had bought an unlucky diamond. This incident remained an unsolved mystery in the author's mind until the allergy to diamonds was encountered in the previous case. Maybe the mystery has been solved!

A 44-year-old woman came to the office complaining of severe pain in the left thigh, left knee, and below the knee all the way to the ankle joint. She had the pain for a year and three months. During that time, she had seen two neurologists, an orthopedic doctor, a chiropractor and a rolfer. She took massages at least once a week hoping that would increase the circulation and get rid of the pain. She had to go to the emergency room four times during this time, due to excruciating pain that she could not control with the pain pills, and she had to get a pain shot. She was a social drinker and never used any drugs or tobacco, other than the pain pills she was taking for the continuous nagging muscle spasm of the leg. Her X-rays and other examinations were perfectly normal, except for mild osteoporotic signs on the bones. She was taking hormone therapy to reduce the presumed osteoporosis.

In our office, she was evaluated thoroughly via her history, physical examination, etc., including allergy tests for foods, chemicals, and environmental materials. She showed a high allergy to metals. She was wearing a huge diamond stone ring on her left finger. When she was tested for the diamonds, she was found to be highly allergic to them, and it was also found by kinesiological examination that the allergy was localized on the left leg. At that time she said that she was wearing another large diamond ring on the right hand when she went to dinner. She also recalled that she was a polio victim as a child, and her left leg was the affected limb even though she is now completely recovered.

Upon questioning her further, it was discovered that she got these two diamond rings from her husband when she was married, a year and four months earlier. Soon after the marriage, she was sick with a severe bladder infection and flu-like symptoms for three weeks. When she recovered from the infection, she developed the muscle spasm and pain in the leg. The pain and discomfort of her leg went away when she was treated for the diamond by Nambudripad's Allergy Elimination Techniques.

From some of these case studies, the reader can understand how much the electromagnetic energies of substances can influence the health of humans (and probably other living beings) and cause energy blockages. We spoke of their adverse affects on the body. Let us consider the possible chances of good effects. Let us take the example of the diamond stone with the strong electromagnetic energy.

If the energy of the diamond is perceived as compatible by the brain, the energy from the diamond would add to the body's energy and enhance the energy flow through the meridians. This strengthened energy might even help remove possible energy blockages, leading to better health for the wearer. Many people believe in wearing birthstones for health, happiness and success. This may explain why it is a possibility. However, compatibility with the stone is absolutely necessary for positive enhancement of energy, as we have just seen in the case of the woman's problems with the unlucky or unsuitable diamond. Likewise, if one is surrounded by a lot of suitable energy fields from many different items in a room, the energy from all the products will flow through the person and he will feel energetic and happy, because as the energy pathways open wide for free flowing energy to circulate through the body without any obstruction. This would in turn improve the blood and nutrients circulation. All the cells and tissues of the body will be well supplied with plenty of oxygen and nutrients. This will make the person healthy and happy.

On the other hand, if one is surrounded by unsuitable charges from many objects around him that cause energy blockages in his meridians at various parts of the body, no matter how much one tries to help him with massages, therapies and medications, his discomfort would only increase and no relief will be in sight.

In the case of the above described 48 year old newlyweds, the reason for her illness soon after the wedding was very likely the powerful negative affect of the diamonds. A diamond has one of the strongest energy fields and her lower limb was already weak due to the previous polio infection. Blockages always start at the weakest area of the body.

A unique case is worth mentioning here. A 24 year old woman met a man and was married two weeks later. They moved to a different state. Her husband was very much into clean living and good eating habits. He used only complex carbohydrates and unprocessed foods. This was something new for her, a girl with a little sophistication in that area. A couple of weeks after their marriage, she became very ill. She had chronic bronchitis that did not settle down with antibiotics. She complained of severe body aches in all her joints all of the time. She felt depressed and also suffered from severe insomnia. Her concerned husband took her from doctor to doctor in the hope of getting his wife some relief.

One of the doctors asked her what made her better or worse. Her answer was that she felt better when she had her husband's arm around her. That was the only time she felt relief from her pain. At all other times, she hurt in spite of taking many aspirin or Tylenol pills a day. The doctor shook his head and referred her to a psychiatrist for the treatment of psychosomatic ailments. The psychiatrist agreed with her previous doctor and advised her to go to Hawaii or some such place for a vacation. He thought she was seeking more attention from her husband. They tried the vacation and went to Hawaii and Tahiti for a few weeks, but her condition remained the same.

It turned out that she was allergic to all the health foods and unprocessed foods. She was highly allergic to the B-complex family, which made her allergic to all the foods that contained B-complex vitamins. When she started eating whole wheat products on a high fiber diet, her body started building up toxins that caused her all that physical and mental agony. Nobody suspected the cause of the problems to have been allergies. She was not allergic to her husband nor was he to her. When she sat next to him, his strong energy field was enhanced and added to her own energy, improved her energy circulation, and temporarily removed any blockages. That is why she felt better in contact with him. The lady now lives a happy, healthy life with her husband and a nine year old son.

Wouldn't it be wonderful if a simple test could be taught allergy sufferers that could detect and predetermine the potentially harmful reactions between substances and people before adverse electromagnetic energies create havoc in their systems, bringing on ill health and unhappiness?

We have been able to do just that after many years of research. We can manipulate our brains and nervous systems to our desires and for our benefit. We can reprogram our brains to accept unsuitable energies as suitable ones and use them for our benefit, rather than allow them to cause energy blockages and imbalances. We do not have to hide from certain food items that we like the most. We do not have to throw away our favorite clothes because they make us sick. We do not have to hide indoors during the pollen season. We do not have to spend the rest of our days in metropolitan areas instead of vacationing in the mountains, because of fear of poison oak and mosquitoes. We do not have to look pale, sick and aged instead of using the latest cosmetic products that would make us look at least 20 years younger, because of fear of skin rashes and hives. We do not have to hide from sunny beaches for fear of skin problems and skin cancers. We do not have to end up in divorce courts soon after the marriages that we thought would last forever. We could even avoid seeing our teenagers using drugs and alcohol, finally ending up in suicides, if we were able to uncover the problems in time, before they take over lives.

Our psychiatric hospitals might not be filled with overflowing mentally ill people, if we could only find the causes of our energy blockages and remove them. Our county jails would not be packed as full as they are now, if inmates' allergies were found and treated. We might be able to prevent heart attacks and other tragic deaths, due to cancer and other "incurable" diseases, if we could teach the whole world to find their suitable electromagnetic fields, stick to them, and avoid unsuitable energy from a very early age or use Nambudripad's Allergy Elimination Techniques to change the unsuitable energies to suitable ones. If everyone learned and practiced these techniques from childhood on, we might be able to stop many disease processes, perhaps even postpone the aging process.

These successful, 100% effective Nambudripad's Allergy Elimination Techniques are available to the whole world. It is up to professionals to learn them and use them on their patients, and it is up to the public to get them from their doctors and get the full benefit of this new, remarkably effective treatment method.

PART II

**NAMBUDRIPAD'S ALLERGY
ELIMINATION TECHNIQUES:
A REVOLUTIONARY APPROACH**

CHAPTER EIGHT

THE BIRTH OF NAMBUDRIPAD'S ALLERGY ELIMINATION TECHNIQUES

Allergic conditions occur much more commonly than one realizes. To get an idea of the number of people suffering from allergies, and of how frequently the allergic condition occurs, one has only to visit a large multi-function clinic in the area. A large proportion of the total number of patients will be in the allergy clinic.

Every year there are more and more recognized cases of allergy. There are probably two reasons for this. The first is that physicians are becoming more allergy conscious and are, therefore, recognizing and diagnosing them more frequently. The second is that due to the large increase in population in our large cities; where certain industrial dust, chemicals, fumes, environmental pollutants, pollens, etc., are proliferating, more people develop allergic symptoms. We live in a chemical, technological age where researchers and scientists are competing with each other every minute of the day to get better products into the marketplace. Hence, new products are being created every day.

The continuous discovery of various chemical compounds being used to manufacture articles of everyday use, including clothing and fabrics, creates new allergens and many people quickly develop a sensitivity to them. It is estimated that 90 percent of the population suffers from allergies. In some instances the reactions are predictable, but for others the reactions are not predictable. They vary radically and appear unexpectedly, making diagnoses elusive and pre-treatments nearly impossible.

For those whose lives are merely disrupted by the discomfort of the reaction, simple antihistamine or topical remedies bring

111

temporary relief until the season passes. But for those whose lives are being threatened, long-term immunotherapy or complete avoidance is the only hope the medical field has been able to offer so far. This, of course is very expensive, and time consuming and often does not present a very satisfactory outcome. Most people finally resort to a lifetime of depriving themselves of many of the things in life that bring them joy and fulfillment. Common complaints are, "My allergies have taken control of my life," and, "The very best things that I want to make me happy are the very things that I react to the most."

Even with total isolation from potential allergens, there is no guarantee that allergy sufferers will be able to stay away from every situation and keep reaction free. New products are being developed every day that are essential allergens. With the progress of science and technology the lifestyle of mankind has changed very much, and the quality of life has also improved. But for some allergic patients, the scientific achievements have turned into everlasting nightmares.

For the purpose of an introduction to this new method of treatment for people suffering from allergies, a thorough treatise on biochemistry is not appropriate. Instead, the discussion will concentrate on the basic ideas around which it is constructed and give some insight into the lives of the people whom it has helped. This is not a new technology. It is actually a combination of techniques, using much of what is already known from chiropractic, kinesiology and acupuncture. Doctor Devi S. Nambudripad; who is a registered nurse, a chiropractor, a kinesiologist, and an acupuncturist, did many years of research and experimentation in these three fields of healing techniques. She came up with a combination of techniques to eliminate energy blockages and to restore the body to a healthy state. These energy blockage elimination techniques are called "Nambudripad's Allergy Elimination Technique."

The energy blockages in the human body are caused by unsuitable charges around the body. When there is an unsuitable charge around the body, there is an altered reaction in the body. This type of energy incompatibility or energy blockage that is capable of producing various ailments is used synonymously with "allergy" in this book.

It is important to recognize that allergies do not exist in a vacuum. They are a part of a complex interrelation between the allergen and the central nervous system, which controls the proper function of the various organs, and the digestive, skeletal, vascular, and lymphatic system. Each of these complex systems, under the direction of the central nervous system, is capable of ignoring or reacting to a given stimulus. This happens either in concert with all other systems, producing a massive shut down of the human machine, or producing weakness and malfunction of any of the parts of the total system.

The exact reason the central nervous system chooses to react to or ignore a given stimulus on any occasion is not known so far. There are large areas of the brain still under investigation for their function. One area which has been dramatically observed is that severe asthmatics do not experience attacks when they are frightened. In these situations, the body prepares for "fight or flight." In this "hyperchemical" state, the allergens are totally ignored. The adjustment has been made as surely as though a switch had been thrown. The author utilized this idea when she developed Nambudripad's Allergy Elimination Techniques as a treatment to permanently eliminate allergies. Each time a person is treated for an allergen, a temporary "fight or flight" reaction is created in the body, which is forced to create the appropriate chemical and make the proper adjustment in the presence of the allergen. During the hyperchemical state once again the allergen is totally ignored and, at a future time, whenever that particular allergen comes in contact with the body, the body automatically goes into a hyperchemical state and does not react to the allergen any more.

An allergenic substance may not produce the same kind of result in every individual. Let us compare the different reactions of eight people to a common allergen such as chocolate. In each case, the standard scratch test and blood serum analysis did not identify chocolate as an allergen for that patient.

Case 1:   Patient exhibited hyperactivity and insomnia upon eating chocolate.

Case 2:   Patient's symptoms were acute asthmatic distress.

Case 3:   Chocolate resulted in vascular headache approaching the magnitude of migraines.

Case 4:   Patient experienced extreme tiredness and unable to keep awake.

Case 5:   Whenever the patient ate chocolate, she became extremely emotional and often depressed.

Case 6:   Patient experienced severe indigestion, bloating, and belching.

Case 7:   Patient had severe pain in the joints of the extremities, similar to that of arthritis.

Case 8:   Patient had severe diarrhea minutes after she consumed chocolate.

Most of these patients, in spite of the medical test results to the contrary, knew by instinct and experience that they should not eat chocolate. How the body reacted to contact with the allergen was not consistent with every patient. Rather, each patient's body reacted at the perverse whim of the central nervous system.

The expression of the allergic reaction seemed to be centered in one or more of the organs alerted to the presence of the substance, in or near the body. The observation is consistent with traditional Oriental medicine, which holds that treatment for most diseases should begin with making adjustments to the central nervous system, the center of the balance between all other bodily functions. Offending elements introduced into the system trigger imbalances. This adversely affects the essence of the body or "qi," further manifesting the problem in pathology of the various tissues and organs, or the "Zang Fu."

The pathology can then be clearly demonstrated, first as a kinetic weakness, observable through standard muscle response testing techniques from applied kinesiology. In fact, each of the chocolate allergy sufferers mentioned above exhibited weakness when given a muscle response test. This fact then becomes the pivotal premise in the foundation of "Nambudripad's Allergy Elimination Techniques" therapy model. Kinetic or muscle weakness makes diagnosis possible. Muscle weakness is the body's way of signaling the patient and the doctor about potential negative reactions to allergens. Since a simple and effective diagnostic tool is now available, it becomes a matter of good detective work to identify all the substances that may be responsible for the symptoms.

When Oriental medicine was introduced to the Western world some decades ago, many Western medical minds were amazed that many so called psychosomatic illnesses responded nicely to acupuncture treatment. They were even more amazed when they began to unlock the secrets of the central nervous system and how it controls the body's functioning, including all organs.

They also knew that by stimulating the trunk of the central nervous system, and its branches or meridians that form the complex link between the brain and various body parts, one could effect temporary relief from pain. Although they did not understand the reason, they just developed their methods to benefit their patients.

We do not have to follow the Chinese theory every step of the way, but we could adapt the best of what Chinese medicine can offer and combine it with the best of what Western science can render to us. Putting two knowledges together will be like putting two heads together in solving a problem. These two outstanding medical disciplines should definitely nurture our need to understand ourselves and our brain functions. Yes, we could help ourselves and solve a lot of mysterious, "incurable" health problems by learning to strengthen our brain and nervous system.

As stated earlier, all living and nonliving substances as well as the earth have a magnetic energy around them. All these substances are attracted to the earth by the earth's magnetic energy. That is why all of us stay grounded on the earth instead of flying in space. Similarly, all the substances on the surface also are attracted to each other by each item's own magnetic force. We all are products of the same universe, so we all are interrelated with each other. This may have been the state of the world when it began. Over the years, due to genetic mutation, genes of all living things have changed slightly, or altered, from the original creation mainly due to replication. Replication usually creates differences in any items. Some are noticeable and some are not.

When humans are replicated, the genes are altered from time to time depending upon the time and circumstances of the replication. That is why children may not look like parents in most cases. If some of the energy channels were blocked during the time of replication or during the transfer of the genetic message, the reproduced gene will carry all the messages except the blocked area. When this partial replication is repeated over and over, transferred genes may perhaps lose the ability to recognize certain items that cause the blockage during the time of replication. In other words, the brain does not have the ability to recognize some of the energies around it, and what it does not recognize, it starts to repel.

From this assumption, we can form another hypothesis. Allergic sensitivities are nothing but the signals to the central nervous system gone awry. The product of these signals, which create repulsion between the central nervous system and other substances, have little to do with the toxic or nontoxic properties of the substances. Instead, they are the result of the way the central nervous system perceives the substance and decides whether it is a compatible field or not.

In other words, it is nontoxic or toxic according to how the brain perceives it. If it is perceived as toxic, it will cause blockages in the energy channels, if nontoxic, it will aid the energy flow in the channels helping to clear any blockage present. The extent of the clearance will depend upon the strength of the compatible field of the substance. This bring us to the concept, which is revolutionary to most people. "Allergic reactions are the result of a message received and acted upon by the central nervous system and are not the result of the inherent properties of the substances we come in contact with."

The quest of every patient and, indeed, the whole medical profession, is to solve the riddle that will change the signals from "danger" to "harmless." Of course, each medical philosophy has developed its own treatment concepts and each has its own following. The adherents of each philosophy clings to his or her particular treatment modalities and procedures, tenaciously directing patients to attain whatever levels of healing are possible through them.

Still, at best, real relief and comfort come only when total avoidance of the allergens is possible. And even then, as is often the case, new allergies replace those that are successfully avoided, leaving the patient as bad off or worse than before. So the question still remains, "Is a permanent cure possible for allergies?" Can the central nervous system, which has been conditioned to respond in rebellion against the body for a long time, perhaps for millennia, be reprogrammed and brought under submission? Can the central nervous system be trained to send positive signals that can attract anything around it and benefit the body, instead of conflicting with these fields of force and damaging the body balance? Can our own nervous system help us to become free from the damaging effects of allergies? Is a permanent cure for allergies possible? At last the answer to these questions is a definite "yes."

The central nervous system has the ability to ignore or reject a substance's field of force and create a large variety of physical, physiological, and psychological problems in the body, due to its adapted quality or repulsive nature. The same nervous system has the ability to accept or approve certain other forces around us and make us feel good and comfortable. This is because of its acquired ability of attraction from the beginning, before it lost the ability of attraction, due to cell mutation. That means that the brain was aware of the ability of attraction once, and now it has been forgotten. We need to retrain the body to go back to its original function, so we can make the nervous system accept the presence of other rejected items without creating blockages or unpleasantness in the body. This can be accomplished. The treatment produces a permanent result, and the sufferers from allergies will be free at last.

In previous chapters, we have seen that the allergen or adverse charges of a substance can be clearly demonstrated as a kinetic weakness, observable through standard muscle response testing techniques from applied kinesiology. This fact then becomes the pivotal premise in the foundation of Nambudripad's techniques therapy model. Kinetic or muscle weakness makes diagnosis possible.

Can the Nambudripad's Allergy Elimination Techniques offer a solution?

Acupuncture stimulates the central nervous system, provides temporary relief from pain and promotes healing. In the past year, many articles have been written about allergies in publications from holistic and traditional medical writers. In every case, there is a message of hope along with a treatment methodology that includes a strict diet and/or some other careful regimen of behavior. Some of these methods even include one or more of the holistic techniques described above. In every case, there are warnings to the patient about the potential for a relapse if the maintenance doses are not taken or if certain foods are not completely eliminated from the diet. In no instance of treatment is there hope for a total and irreversible cure. They are right to be cautious, because in order to achieve permanent relief from allergic reactions, the central nervous system must be reprogrammed to sense allergens differently than before treatment. The question is, "Is this possible?"

The answer to this question was discovered quite by accident in 1983 by the author, a patient herself, when she was treated by acupuncture for the relief of an allergic reaction to raw carrots. During the treatment, she fell asleep with the carrots still in her hand. After a few minutes of acupuncture treatment, and a restful nap during the needling period, she woke up and experienced a unique feeling which she had never quite felt after other similar acupuncture treatments in the past. Then she realized that she was still holding the carrot in her hand. She knew that some of the needles were supposed to help circulate the electrical energy and balance the body. During the balancing process, if there is any energy blockage it is supposed to clear during the treatment and bring the body to a balanced state. she had studied this concept at school.

She asked her husband, who was assisting her in the treatment process, to test her for carrots again. The carrot's energy field had interacted with her own energy field, and her brain had accepted this once deadly poison as a harmless item, and the two energy fields no longer clashed. This was an amazing NEW DISCOVERY. Subsequent tests for carrots, by muscle response testing, confirmed that something phenomenal had indeed happened. Repeated hourly testing the rest of the day, and eating carrots the next day without any allergic reaction, confirmed the result. Her central nervous system had learned a different response to the stimulus, and she was no longer reactive to it.

In some mysterious way, the treatment had reprogrammed the brain. What followed was a series of experiments treating the author's own allergies and those of her family. She cured all her allergies in a year's time. The method was finally extended to her practice. In every case, allergies were "cleared out," never to return. After treating thousands of patients, for a wide variety of allergies, the procedure is no longer experimental and of questionable value. It is a proven treatment method and the premise of Nambudripad's Allergy Elimination Technique's methodology.

Physical contact with the allergen during and after a treatment (which consists of stimulating certain specific points on the acupuncture meridians, thus stimulating the central nervous system), produces the necessary immune mediators or antidotes to neutralize the adverse reaction coming from the allergen in the hand. This produces a totally new, permanent and irreversible response to the allergen. It is possible, through stimulation of the appropriate points of the acupuncture meridians that have direct correspondence with the brain, to reprogram the brain.

The success of the Nambudripad's Allergy Elimination Techniques procedure confirms that a major portion of the illnesses we observe result from allergies. This includes the experience of a 65-year-old man who complained of a hacking cough during the day, but not when he went to bed at night. It was found that he was allergic to the cough drops he used to chew during the day. It also includes the 5-day-old infant with the cardiac arrhythmia (a rapid and irregular heartbeat without any physical heart problem) which occurred after feeding. It was discovered he was allergic to his mother's milk.

For people like the 11-year-old Little League baseball player who accidentally ate a cookie made with peanuts and died within minutes from allergy produced shock, this breakthrough in treatment technique is too late. But for many others, the prognosis is bright. The treatment procedure has already been used to help another Little League player who had reacted much the same way to a rice cereal. Testing assures his parents that this boy will never have to worry about an accidental encounter with the once deadly rice cereal filled snack after a baseball game. And what would the prognosis be for the little girl who was the victim of a similar accidental allergic poisoning from peanuts, which resulted in stroke and in coma and paralysis for three months. If she had not been given a long series of Nambudripad's Allergy Elimination Techniques treatment for the specific type of peanut butter that had been used in the cookie she ate at her friend's house, would she be walking around today a bright, happy and hope filled? Undoubtedly not.

Yes, the prognosis is bright. A convincing argument can be made that a significant number of patients suffering from latent, undiagnosed allergies normally treated by traditional medical practitioners for temporary relief are going to experience a cure from holistic health practitioners. Freedom from allergies, or SAY GOOD-BYE TO ILLNESS is becoming a fact for many patients presenting a wide range of symptoms, from chemical dependency and stroke, to eczema and asthma.

This is an age of instant solutions to everything and medicine is no exception. We helped design the system, as it now exists, by our insistence on instant cures to our discomforts. We want to be well, and we want to be well now! We suffer from a syndrome that says, "I don't care how much the medication costs as long as it will make me feel better in a couple of minutes." Then we are disappointed when we have to wait for months and years to get relief and, in most cases, never ever get a relief. It is no wonder then, that patients are not prepared to take charge of their own health care. They have not learned what it means to be informed enough to be in charge.

So, the first lesson to be learned about taking charge of our own health care is to be informed, not only about our obvious health care needs, but about the processes that take place within the body that result in poor health. When a person is chronically ill and symptoms persist or recur, shortly after being treated and after completing medications, the patient must learn as much as possible about the problem. He or she must make an effort to make decisions about health care alternatives.

The public should be educated, particularly in these instances, that allergies should not be dismissed lightly as a possible root cause of these seemingly incurable or recurring symptoms. The public should be educated in how to find the cause of their problem. If the problem could be traced, they could easily avoid the contact with the causative agent. If the contact is unavoidable, they could go to any of the medical professionals who have learned to eliminate the problem using Nambudripad's Allergy Elimination Techniques.

Hundreds of doctors of allopathic, chiropractic, osteopathy, dentistry and acupuncture all over the United States, Canada, Europe and other countries have been trained to treat effectively with this new revolutionary technique. Regular training sessions are being conducted many times a year to prepare more licensed doctors of allopathy, chiropractic, acupuncture and osteopathy to meet the challenge. This book will educate individuals to test themselves and locate the cause of their problem. Steps of treatments are not given here, because that is beyond the scope of this book. The information about the training is available for the qualified doctors and given at the back of this book.

CHAPTER NINE

ACUPUNCTURE MERIDIANS

ENERGY PATHWAYS

The human body is made up of bones, flesh, nerves, and blood vessels, all of which have very important functions. Each of these can only function in the presence of vital energy. Without this energy, the body is like an advanced efficient computer without an electrical power supply. Vital energy is not visible to the human eye, however, neither is electricity. No one knows how or why the vital energy gets into the body or how, when or where it goes when it leaves. It is true, however, that without vital energy, none of the body functions can take place. When the vital energy flows freely through the meridians or energy pathways, the human body is said to be alive. When this takes place the blood will begin to circulate through the blood vessels and distribute appropriate nutrients into the various parts of the body.

The blood will also help to exchange oxygen and carbon dioxide, thus cleaning up the impurities of the body. When it gets proper nutrients, the body and bones will grow, and the flesh and nerves will protect the body. All the body parts will work as a unit, and all the functions will go on as scheduled like an efficient factory. When vital energy stops to flow through the energy pathways, the human machine ceases to function and the person is said to be dead.

The human body is the most efficient, well-organized functional unit ever seen. Each and every cell (the basic building block) of the body is connected with every other cell by many branches of channels and collaterals of energy pathways. In turn, each part of the body is connected and interlinked by a meshing of networks of channels and collaterals, creating a perfect communication system within the body. The brain is the commander of this system. When the vital energy activates this system, the brain takes over the responsibilities. Under the brain's command, all parts of the body are activated and there is open communication between the brain, cells and other body parts. This communication takes place within seconds, thus the brain maintains complete control of the body functions.

If for some reason blockage takes place in the energy pathways, the normal physiology is disrupted. This energy disruption will lead to certain visible effects in the human body, thus, pathological symptoms will begin to appear. These pathological symptoms will be noticed around the blockage(s) in the beginning, and then will spread along the channels and collaterals, related tissues and organs, and finally may affect the whole body.

Acupuncture meridians, or energy pathways, are located throughout the body. They contain a free-flowing, colorless, noncellular liquid. There are many specific acupuncture points along these meridians. Most of them connect or interlink with branches from other meridians. These points are electromagnetic in character and consist of small, oval cells, called Bonham corpuscles. These corpuscles surround the capillaries under the skin, the blood vessels and organs throughout the body. The Chinese have named these meridians by the life functions with which they seem to be associated. In most cases, these names are similar to the names of organs with which we are familiar. Careful study of the course of the channels, and a knowledge of the most commonly seen pathological symptoms, might help the reader to isolate the specific area of the specific meridian that has a blockage. Energy blockage in the respective organs gives rise to specific symptoms that are unique to those meridians. Allergens can block a meridian at three levels: physical, nutritional, chemical or emotional.

PHYSICAL BLOCKAGE

Traditional pathology distinguishes symptoms appearing along the external course of the channels from those affecting internal organs associated with the channels. By studying these symptoms, the blocked areas of the meridians can be identified. Physical blockages can be removed by manual manipulation, massages, simple acupuncture treatments, etc.

A woman, age 54, came in with a severe stiffness and pain in the neck which began when she woke in the morning. Kinesiological testing revealed that she had vegetables of some kind the previous night that caused this stiff neck. Upon further questioning, it was discovered that she had green beans for dinner. Bean allergy caused physical problems for her. If she had been treated with chiropractic, or straight needles, physical therapy, massage, or even with some pain pills, she would have received relief in couple of days. Since we knew her problem was due to green beans, she was treated for beans with NAET, and she became symptom free in less than 10 minutes.

NUTRITIONAL BLOCKAGE

Nutritional or chemical blockages affect mainly the internal pathways of acupuncture meridians. These types of blockages can be removed effectively by using NAET techniques. The chemical or nutritional level blockages can give rise to acute or chronic allergic symptoms. Acute allergic symptoms are felt by the patients with in 24 hours of coming in contact with the allergens. Chronic allergic symptoms are felt after 24 hours of exposure with the allergens.

A man age 32 had complaints of instant runs to the bathroom as soon as he took a bite of egg products. He could cook for others and touch the egg or chicken without any problems. He was treated for eggs by NAET. Now he eats as many eggs as he wants, with out any digestive problems.

EMOTIONAL BLOCKAGE

Allergens can cause energy blockages at the emotional aspect of the meridian. This can also be treated very effectively using NAET techniques. Emotional allergies also can be treated by psychiatrists, and psychologists using traditional treatments and therapies.

A woman, age 45, was brought into the office, accompanied by her husband, about 9 a.m. She was holding a basin under her chin and appeared to be nauseated. Upon questioning, her husband revealed her history. She began throwing up about 8 p.m. the night before, soon after she ate a peach. Her abdomen was very distended. She was unable to urinate, move her bowels or pass flatus the whole night. She was unable to keep anything in the stomach due to vomiting, and complained of a knot at the solar plexus. Her husband took her to the emergency room about 5 a.m. in the morning. She went through a series of tests, and radiological examination showed that she had an intestinal obstruction. She was advised to go to surgery to remove the obstruction. She was familiar with our treatment methods, since she has had many treatments for migraines and a few other complaints in our office.

When the emergency room doctor suggested surgery, she immediately thought of us and asked her husband to bring her to our clinic. By this time the patient was getting very weak, her pulse was weak and thready, her skin was cold and clammy and she was perspiring profusely. To keep her from fainting, a few acupuncture needles were inserted on selected points. She was too weak to do any tests at that point. Her husband was used as a surrogate to do the tests. With the help of kinesiology, her problem was traced to an emotional blockage from peach that happened about 8 p.m. last night. When the words emotional blockage were mentioned, her husband narrated the following story. Her 17-year-old son was on a cross country tour and he was on phone with her from New Hampshire about 8 p.m. last night. In the middle of the conversation, the connection got disturbed, she heard some loud noises and gunshots. The phone went dead. She suddenly came to a conclusion that somebody had shot her son and killed him. She was holding a half-eaten peach in her hand while talking to him on the phone.

The allergy to peach was found to be the cause of her intestinal obstruction. It was further simplified as an emotional allergy to peach. While she got frightened with the cutoff phone conversation and gunshot sounds, her confused brain did not have enough time to sort out the matters. The brain probably took it for granted that eating peach was the cause of her fear and unhappiness at that time and continued to caution her from getting peach into her stomach. She was immediately treated for emotion peach allergy by NAET. In two minutes, her ailing body became alive again. She was able to breathe with out pain, her color came back, her body became warm and dry, and she was not nauseated anymore. She drank some water without a problem. She was able to urinate instantly, which relieved the distention of the abdomen. Her dramatic instantaneous recovery from a possible surgery amazed not only she and her husband but, also the office staff.

By the way, her son was calling her from a public telephone and the area was too noisy and the line got cut off. After he reached his hotel room he had called home again to let them know that everything was O.K. By this time her brain was misguided by the wrong ideas. In this case, knowing of his safety alone was not enough to assure her brain of removal of the danger.

RELATED MUSCLES

Meridians, their channels, sub-channels and/or collaterals (various branches), travel through various routes in the body including various muscles and tissues. Therefore, the effect of the blockage can also be felt at the muscles and tissues. Each meridian is thus capable of affecting a group of muscles in the body. The weakness or strength of the particular muscle can also give information about the status or integrity of the particular meridian.

A 32-year-old woman suffered from dull, constant pain on her lateral part of the left thigh for five years. The tensor facia lata muscle was just under the area of her said pain. Tensor facia lata is related to the large intestine meridian. She did not have any other complaints. She was married 5 years ago. She was found to be allergic to gold, and the gold caused energy blockages in the large intestine meridian. The blockage of the large intestine meridian was felt as a dull pain on the related muscle tensor facia lata. When the allergy of the gold was eliminated, the pain on the muscle relieved.

TIME

An energy molecule takes 24 hours to travel through the body and to complete the full circulation through all 12 major meridians, branches and sub-branches. It takes two hours to travel through one meridian. According to Oriental medical principles, the qi follows the flow of meridian. The flow begins at the lung meridian and takes two hours to complete it's journey. Likewise, each meridian gets two hours for the energy molecule to pass through. Each meridian gets two hours during the day. Each particular meridian is very strong during its meridian time. If one looks at the two-hour meridian time, then the meridian is at its strongest at the beginning of its meridian time and less effective toward the end of its time.

How does this information affect the allergy treatments? When the allergy is eliminated through NAET, the patient has to wait 24 hours to let the energy molecule carrying the new information to pass through the complete cycle of the journey. If the allergen has caused blockages in one or two meridians, when the energy molecule passes through those affected meridians without disturbance, the patient may not experience adverse symptoms or undo the treatment as the molecule passes through other unblocked meridians. This holds true even if the patient did not observe the avoidance of the allergen for 24 hours.

DENTAL CONNECTION

Some of the small branches of the major meridians pass the gum and dental area. This knowledge helps us to understand why certain teeth hurt or get diseased when eating certain food or when coming in contact with certain chemicals, etc. When a particular tooth gives any discomfort, one should test the related major meridian and organ for certain allergy. Immediate correction of that particular allergy and strengthening of that particular meridian may save you a trip to the dentist or unnecessary, painful, time consuming and expensive dental work.

NUTRITIONAL NEEDS OF THE MERIDIAN

Meridians are part of our body. Our body is made up of flesh, bones and blood; so are the meridians. Our body needs proper nutrition for growth and development and to repair wear and tear. So do the meridians, their related organs and tissues. When one is allergic to nutritional elements, one cannot absorb or utilize the nutrition from the food being eaten. Thus, the body suffers nutritional deficiencies. After the person goes through the allergy elimination treatment, one needs to take nutritious products to eliminate the deficiencies in the body. One needs to supplement, with appropriate nutritional supplements, to strengthen appropriate meridian or related organs and tissues.

If the blocked areas and the causative agents can be identified at a stage of a disease processes (blockage), the cause can be eliminated easily and the energy blockage can be removed immediately. Thus, the human body can be protected from any possible major pathology.

Traditional Chinese medicine describes the meridians, or energy pathways, in detail in the literature as well as the symptomatology of each of the primary channels and secondary channels. In this chapter each of the 12 primary channels, their distribution and symptomatology will be discussed, according to the levels of blockages. Overcharged and underactive energy pathways can also cause health problems. Meridian balancing can solve that problem.

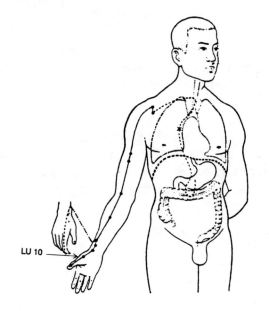

LU 10

Figure 9-1. Lung Channel

LUNG CHANNEL

This channel begins in the region of the stomach (middle burner or warmer) and passes downward to connect with the large intestine. Returning, it follows the cardiac orifice, crosses the diaphragm, and enters its associated organ, the lung. Emerging transversely from the area between the lung and throat, the channel descends along the anterior aspect of the upper arm, lateral to the heart and pericardium channels. Reaching the elbow, it continues along the anterior aspect of the forearm to the anterior margin of the styloid at the wrist. From here it crosses the radial artery at the pulse, and extends over the thenar eminence to the radial side of the tip of the thumb.

A branch splits from the main channel above the styloid process at the wrist and travels directly to the radial side of the tip of the index finger. This channel is associated with the lung and connects with the large intestine. It crosses the diaphragm and is joined with the stomach, the kidney and other organs.

Symptoms associated with the external course of the channel include: congestion; headache; pain in the chest, clavicle, shoulder and back; and chills and pains along the channel of the arm.

Symptoms associated with the internal organ (lung) include coughing, asthma, shortness of breath, fullness in the chest, parched throat, changes in the color of urine, irritability, blood in the sputum, hot palms, sometimes accompanied by distended abdomen and loose stools.

OVERCHARGED OR UNDERACTIVE MERIDIANS

Typical symptoms of an overcharged Lung meridian are heaviness of the chest, short of breath, heavy coughing, and a lot of mucus. In the underactive condition, the patient can have a low immune system, feels like coming down with a cold, frequent sneezing, sniffles, cough, and chills.

ACUTE ALLERGIC SYMPTOMS

Acute symptoms associated with partial or full blockage of the lung meridian include nasal congestion, itching of the nostrils, sneezing, shortness of breath, cough, acute bronchial asthmatic attacks, postnasal drips, mucus in the throat, burning in the nostrils, burning in the eyes, throat irritation, dry mouth, dry throat, sore throat, nose bleed, fever, red or painful eyes, fatigue, insomnia, restlessness, lethargy, flu-like symptoms, frontal headache, maxillary sinus headaches, general body ache, itching of the scalp, itching of the body, generalized urticaria, itching on the course of the lung meridian, pain in the thumb, pain in the course of the lung meridian, dry skin, scaly skin, pain in the first interphalangeal joint, tenosynovitis, pain in the intercostal area, pain in the upper back, runny nose with clear discharge, pain in the upper first cuspid, and second upper bicuspid, chest congestion, pain in the chest, clavicle, pain between third and fourth thoracic vertebrae, pain in the anterior fontanel and pain in the arms and hair loss.

CHRONIC ALLERGIC SYMPTOMS

Symptoms of chronic conditions of lung channel include chronic cough, asthma, shortness of breath, fullness in the chest, influenza, sore throat, runny nose with thick yellow or white drainage, swollen cervical glands, irritability, bronchitis, pneumonia, pleurisy, other chest infections, tuberculosis, blood in the sputum, hot palms, distended abdomen, loose stools, general body ache, insomnia, restlessness, husky voice, arthritis of the thumb, tennis elbow, frozen shoulder, tendinitis on the shoulder, tenosynovitis, pain in the first interphalangeal joint, hair loss, poor growth of hair, emphysema, atopic dermatitis, skin rashes, chronic skin problems, nasal polyps, chronic toothache of upper cuspid and upper second bicuspids.

EMOTIONAL PATTERNS

Lung meridian dysfunction usually evolves from a childhood experience with an older person, a parent, older sibling, a guardian or some one else who repeatedly bossed the child around and criticized the thoughts and opinions of the child. If the child learns to fight back the authority figure, whether cognitively or verbally, an overcharged lung meridian can develop into adulthood. If the child gives up the fight and accepts the bullying authority, then an undercharged lung meridian will be the outcome.

Some of the other commonly observed clinical symptoms of lung meridian blockage at the emotional level are over sympathy, intolerance, over demanding, always apologizing, false pride, contempt, prejudice, meanness, hopelessness, despair, loneliness, dejection, grief, melancholy, depression, self pity, liking to humiliate or insult others, seeking other's approval in doing things, comparing self with others, having low self-esteem, craving sugars, liking pungent and spicy foods, liking onion, peppers, garlic, cinnamon, and weeping frequently without much reason.

RELATED MUSCLES

Serratus anterior, coracobrachialis, deltoids, diaphragm.

RELATED TIME: 3 - 5 a.m.

DENTAL CONNECTION

Upper cuspid, second upper cuspid.

NUTRITION

Clear water, proteins, vitamin C, bioflavonoids, cinnamon, onions, garlic, B-2, citrus fruits, green peppers, black peppers, and rice.

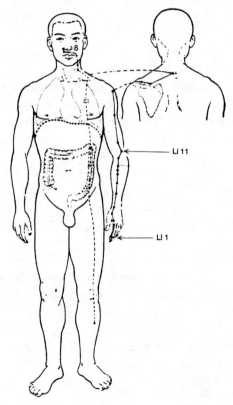

Figure 9-2. Large Intestine Channel

135

LARGE INTESTINE CHANNEL

This channel begins at the radial side of the tip of the index finger and proceeds upward between the first and second metacarpal bones of the hand. It then passes between the tendons of the extensor pollicus longus and brevis at the wrist and continues along the radial margin of the forearm to the lateral side of the elbow. From here it rises along the lateral aspect of the upper arm to the shoulder, following the anterior margin of the acromion, before turning upward. Just beneath the spinous process of the seventh cervical vertebra, the channel enters directly into the supraclavicular fossa and connects with the lung, before descending across the diaphragm to the large intestine.

A branch separates from the main channel at the supraclavicular fossa and moves upward through the neck, crosses the cheek and cheers the lower gum. From here it curves around the lip and intersects the same channel, coming from the opposite side of the body at the philtrum. The branch finally terminates at the side of the nose.

Another branch descends to the stomach at acupuncture point St 37 (Shang Ju Xu), the lower uniting point of the large intestine. This channel is associated with the large intestine and connects with the lung. It also joins directly with the stomach.

Symptoms associated with the external course of the channel include fever, parched mouth and thirst, sore throat, nose bleed, toothache, red and painful eyes, swelling of the neck, pain along the course of the channel on the upper arm, pain in the shoulder and shoulder blade, motor impairment of the fingers, pain in the knee, pain in the lateral aspect of the thigh, and swelling of the lateral part of the knee joint.

Symptoms associated with the internal organ (large intestine) include abdominal pain, intestinal noise, loose stools, asthma, chest congestion, shortness of breath, belching, itching of the body, hives, blisters in the lower gum, inflammation of lower gum, pain in the lateral aspect of the leg below the knee joint, pain in the heel, lethargy and sometimes bloody stools, sinus headaches around the eyes and nose.

OVERCHARGED OR UNDERACTIVE MERIDIANS

An overcharged meridian can cause pain in the shoulders, lower abdomen, pain associated with constipation, light-headedness or dizzy spells. An undercharged condition causes intestinal gas and bloated feeling, dry lips, and constipation.

ACUTE ALLERGIC SYMPTOMS

Fever, dry mouth and throat, sore throat, nosebleed, toothache on lateral incisors, first lower and second lower bicuspid, red and painful eyes, swelling of the neck, pain along the course of the channel on the upper arm, pain in the shoulder or shoulder blade, dizziness, constipation, spastic colon, colitis, bow legs, motor impairment of the fingers, pain in the lateral part of the knees, pain in the lateral aspect of the thighs and swelling of the lateral part of the knee joint.

CHRONIC ALLERGIC SYMPTOMS

Abdominal pain, intestinal colic, flatulence, latent asthma, feeling better after a bowel movement, feeling tired after a bowel movement, bad breath, pain in the heel, chest congestion, shortness of breath, belching, itching of the body, hives, rashes, dermatitis, acne, warts, hair loss, poor growth of nails and hair, arthritis of shoulder joint, knee joint, index finger, wrist joint and lateral part of the elbow, and hip, pain in the lower back, sciatic pain, muscle spasms of lateral thigh, and knee, blisters in the lower gum, inflammation of the lower gum, pain in the lateral aspect of the leg, below knee joint, pain in the heel, lethargy, bloody stool, sinus headaches around eyes and nose, tenosynovitis, tennis elbow, pain and swelling of the index finger.

EMOTIONAL PATTERNS

Guilt, grief, sadness, seeking sympathy, weeping, crying spells, defensiveness, bothered about the past memory, bad dreams, nightmares, talking in the sleep, rolling restlessly in sleep, and inability to recall dreams.

RELATED MUSCLES

Tensor Facia Lata, Quadratus Lumborum and Hamstrings.

RELATED TIME: 5 - 7 a.m.

DENTAL CONNECTIONS

The Facia Lata is associated with the lower lateral incisor, the quadratus lumborum with the lower first bicuspid, and the hamstrings with the first or second lower bicuspid.

ESSENTIAL NUTRITION

Vitamins A, D, E, C, B complex, especially B-1, wheat, bran, oat bran, yogurt, and roughage.

STOMACH CHANNEL

This channel begins beside the nose, then ascends to the root of the nose where it intersects with the bladder channel. Descending along the lateral side of the nose, it enters the upper gum and joins the governing channel at the philtrum, then circles back around the corner of the mouth, meeting the conception channel at the mental labial groove of the chin. From here it follows the angle of the jaw and runs upward in front of the ear. It proceeds along the hairline until it intersects with the gall bladder channel at gall bladder acupuncture point GB 6 (Xuanli). Finally, it crosses to the middle of the forehead, parallel with the hairline, where it joins the governing channel.

One branch separates from the main channel on the lower jaw and descends along the throat, entering the supraclavicular fossa. From there it travels posteriorly to the upper back, where it meets the governing channel internally at points conception channel acupuncture point Co 13 (Shangwan) and conception channel acupuncture point Co 12 (Zhongwan) before entering its associated organ, the stomach, and communicating with the spleen.

Another vertical branch descends directly from the supra-clavicular fossa along the mammillary line, then passes beside the umbilicus and through the lower abdomen to the inguinal region, where it joins with the vertical branch just described. From here the channel crosses to point stomach acupuncture point St 31 (Biguan) on the anterior aspect of the thigh, and descends directly to the patella. It then proceeds along the lateral side of the tibia to the dorsum of the foot, terminating at the lateral side of the tip of the second toe.

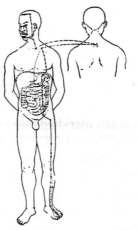

Figure 9-3. Stomach Channel

Another parallel branch separates from the main channel at stomach acupuncture point St 36 (Zunsanli), three units below the knee and terminates at the lateral side of the middle toe. Another branch separates at the dorsum of the foot at stomach acupuncture joint St 42 (Chongyang) and terminates at the medial side of the big toe, where it connects with the Spleen channel at acupuncture point Sp 1 (Yinbai). This channel is associated with the stomach and connects with the spleen. It is also directly joined with the heart, large intestine, and small intestine.

Symptoms associated with the external course of the channel include tidal fever, fever blisters facial paralysis, heat boils, heat boils, black and blue discoloration below the knee.

Symptoms associated with the internal organ (stomach) include: abdominal distension, insomnia, vomiting, nausea, restlessness, mental confusion, personality changes, double personality, obsessive compulsive behaviors, panic disorders, fear of dying, hyperactivity in children or adults, manic-depressive behaviors, lack of concentration, edema, aggressive behaviors, frontal headaches, migraine headaches on the forehead, toothache, pain on the upper jaw and upper gum diseases.

OVERACTIVE AND UNDERACTIVE MERIDIAN

The overactive stomach meridian causes poor or no appetite, unhealthy weight loss, loss of taste, and fatigue. In the overcharged state, the person is overly attentive to the needs and wishes of others. They neglect themselves in the process. They get neglected or abused by others who take advantage of their generosity.

Underactive meridian causes voracious appetite, excess weight and a lot of energy and pain along the stomach channel. The underactive meridian person becomes very selfish, gets involves in self excessive nurturing, etc. Kleptomaniacs fall into this group. A tendency to lie, shop lift, steal, and gamble, are some of the other weaknesses one might see in undercharged groups. They want the best and most comfortable conditions, and the person seems to be out of touch with the needs of others.

ACUTE ALLERGIC SYMPTOMS

High fever, tidal fever, flushed face, sweating, insomnia, delirium, pain in the stomach, nausea, vomiting, sensitivity to cold, pain in the eye, dry nostrils, nosebleed, fever blisters, herpes, sores on the gums and inside of the lips, red painful boils on the face, sore throat, swelling on the neck, facial paralysis, chest pain, hiatal hernia, distention and/or pain along the meridian, fibromyalgia, pain in the leg or foot along the course of the meridian, blood stagnation in the lateral part of the legs, coldness in the lower limbs, acne, heat boils, blemishes, stomatitis, coated tongue, sore tongue, red rashes along the course of the meridian, black and blue discoloration along the channel, especially below the knee, itching on the skin along the channel, pain in the mid-back at the levels of the thoracic vertebrae 6, 8, and 10.

CHRONIC ALLERGIC SYMPTOMS

Abdominal distention, fullness, edema, discomfort while reclining, seizures, persistent hunger, yellow urine, yellow or white thick coat on the tongue, cracks in the center of the tongue, abdominal cramps, vomiting, nausea, anorexia, frontal headache, headaches behind the eyes, dull pain, sharp pain, or pressure pain, burning pain behind the eyes, migraine headaches, insomnia, pain on the upper jaws, temporo-mandibular joint problem, fibromyalgia, upper gum diseases, toothaches, sinus problems, nasal polyps, bad breath, fever blisters, cold sores, tiredness, and insomnia.

EMOTIONAL PATTERNS

Disgust, bitterness, disappointment, greed, emptiness, deprivation, restlessness, obsession, egotism, despair, lack of concentration, nostalgia, mental confusion, mental fogging, manic disorders, schizophrenia, hyperactivity, extreme nervousness, butterfly sensation in the stomach, and aggressive behaviors.

RELATED MUSCLES

Pectoralis major clavicular, brachioradialis, sterno-cleidomastoidus , neck flexors, neck extensors, scalene muscle, levator scapulae.

RELATED TIME: 7 - 9 a.m.

DENTAL CONNECTION

The pectoralis major clavicular is associated with the first and second upper bicuspid. The neck flexors and extensors are connected with the upper central incisors.

ESSENTIAL NUTRITION

B-Complex especially B-12, B-6, B-3 and Folic acid

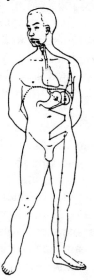

Figure 9-4. Spleen Channel

SPLEEN CHANNEL

This channel begins on the medial tip of the big toe. From here it follows the border between the dark and light skin of the medial aspect of the foot. It then passes in front of the medial malleolus and up the leg, along the posterior side of the tibia, crossing, and then traveling anterior to the liver channel. From here it crosses over the medial aspect of the knee and continues upward along the anterior, medial aspect of the thigh and into the abdomen. Then it crosses the conception channel at acupuncture point Co 3 (Zhongi) and acupuncture point Co 4 (Guanyuan), the channel enters its associated organ, the spleen and communicates with the stomach. It then ascends across the diaphragm and intersects the gall bladder channel at acupuncture point GB24 (Riyue), and the liver channel at acupuncture point Liv 14 (Qimen). Continuing upward beside the esophagus, it crosses the lung channel at acupuncture point Lu 1 (Zhongfu) and finally reaches the root of the tongue dispersing over its lower surface.

A branch of this channel separates in the stomach region and advances upward across the diaphragm, transporting qi into the heart. This channel is associated with the spleen and connects with the stomach. It also directly joins with the heart, lungs, and large intestine.

Symptoms associated with the external course of the spleen channel include heaviness in the body or head, general feverishness, general body ache, fatigued limbs, emaciated muscles, stiffness of the tongue, coldness of the leg and knee along the medial side, edema of the foot and leg, generalized edema of the body, pain in the toes, overweight, sluggishness, lethargy, lack of enthusiasm, lack of interest in anything, moodiness, grumpy nature, and inability to make any decision.

Symptoms associated with the internal organ (spleen) include abdominal pain, fullness or distension, diarrhea, incomplete digestion of food, intestinal noises, nausea, vomiting, lack of taste, lack of smell, hard lumps in the abdomen, reduced appetite, jaundice, constipation, hypoglycemic reaction, pallor, tiredness, sleeplessness, scanty menstrual flow, irregular periods, absence of menstruation, cramps after the first day of menstrual periods, dizzy spells, light-headedness, tingling in the tips of the fingers and palms, carpal tunnel syndrome, pain and stiffness in the interphalangeal joints and wrist joints.

OVERACTIVE AND UNDERACTIVE MERIDIAN

The overactive state causes a person to be extremely indecisive. He continues to swallow new things before the present items are fully digested. This happens with food, job, relationship and many other aspects of life. The overcharged spleen person may acquire a reputation of being extremely fickle.

The underactive state causes craving of sweets, loss of memory, sleepiness during the day, waking up during the night, bouts of depression, withdrawal, hypochondriasis, lack of concentration, forgetfulness, absent mindedness, indifference, difficulty giving and receiving sympathy, difficulty reaching out to new sources, difficulty leaving the old and past behind, and trying to nurture on the past memory.

ACUTE ALLERGIC SYMPTOMS

Heaviness in the body or head, general feverishness, general body aches, fatigued limbs, sugar craving, stiffness of the tongue, coldness of the leg and knee along the medial side, edema of the foot, and leg, generalized edema, generalized body ache, fibromyalgia, pain in the great toes, excess weight, sluggishness, lethargy, lack of enthusiasm, lack of interest in anything, mood swings, grumpy nature, inability to make decision, low self esteem, depression, indigestion, loose stools, and diarrhea, procrastination, sleep during the day, general fatigue, latent insomnia, and dreams that make you tired, intuitive and prophetic behaviors.

CHRONIC ALLERGIC SYMPTOMS

Abdominal pains, fullness or distention, diarrhea, loose stools, undigested food in the stools, incomplete digestion of food, intestinal noises, nausea, vomiting, lack of taste, lack of smell, hard lumps in the abdomen, obesity, diabetes, hypoglycemia, hyperglycemia, sugar craving, general fatigue, chronic fatigue syndromes, retention of fluids in the body especially in the feet, reduced appetite, jaundice, constipation, pallor, scanty menstrual flow, irregular periods, absence of menstruation, cramps after the first day of menses, dizzy spells, light headedness, tingling in the tip of the fingers and palms, carpel tunnel syndrome, fibromyalgia, general body aches, pain and stiffness in the interphalangeal joints and wrist joints, emaciated muscles, weak limbs.

EMOTIONAL PATTERNS

Pensiveness, over concern, worry, low self esteem, lives through others, hopelessness, lack of confidence, over sympathetic to others, gives more importance to self, obsessive compulsive behavior, unable to make decision, shy, timid, restrained, easily hurt, keeps the feelings inside, likes to take revenge, talks to self, likes loneliness, does not like crowds, likes to be praised, and likes to get constant encouragement otherwise falls apart.

RELATED MUSCLES Latissimus dorsi, middle trapezius, triceps, opponens pollicus longus, and lower trapezius.

RELATED TIME: 9 - 11 a.m.

DENTAL CONNECTION The latissimus dorsi is associated with the upper first molar and middle trapezius with the upper third molar.

ESSENTIAL NUTRITION Vitamin A, vitamin C, Calcium, chromium, and protein.

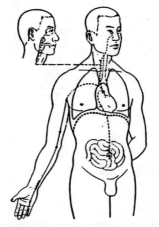

Figure 9-5. Heart Channel

HEART CHANNEL

This channel begins in its associate organ - the heart. Then it emerges through the blood vessel system surrounding the heart and travels downward across the diaphragm, where it connects with the small intestine.

A branch of the main channel separates in the heart and ascends alongside the esophagus to the face, where it joins the tissue surrounding the eye.

Another branch goes directly from the heart to the lung, then slants downward to merge below the axilla. From here the channel descends along the medial border of the anterior aspect of the upper arm, behind the lung and pericardium channels to the ante-cubital fossa where it continues downward to the capitate bone proximal to the palm. It then enters the palm and follows the medial side of the little finger to the finger tip.

147

This channel is associated with the heart and connects with the small intestine. It is also directly joined to the lung and kidneys.

Symptoms associated with the external course of this channel include general feverishness, headache, pain in the eyes, pain along the back of the upper arm, dry throat, hot or painful palms, coldness in the palms and soles of the feet, pain along the scapula or medial aspect of the forearm.

Symptoms associated with the internal organ (heart) include pain or fullness in the chest and ribs or below the ribs, irritability, shortness of breath, discomfort when reclining, vertigo, mental disorders, nervousness, excessive perspiration, insomnia, chest distension, palpitation, sadness, heaviness in the chest, emotional excesses such as excessive laughing or crying, sometimes abusive, sharp chest pain, irregular or knotted pulse, nausea, dizziness, or light-headedness.

OVERACTIVE OR UNDERACTIVE MERIDIAN

The overactive state causes a person to talk a lot, have dry mouth, and heaviness on the chest. The underactive state causes extreme fatigue, and heart palpitation.

ACUTE ALLERGIC SYMPTOMS

General palpitation, dizziness, shoulder pains, chest pains, feverishness, headache, pain in the eye, pain along the heart meridian, poor circulation, dry throat, hot or painful palms, and soles of the feet, pain along the scapula, pain along the medial aspect of the forearm.

CHRONIC ALLERGIC SYMPTOMS

Chest pains, pain and fullness in the chest, ribs, below the ribs, irritability, shortness of breath, discomfort when reclining, vertigo, mental disorders, nervousness, excessive perspiration, insomnia, chest distention, palpitation, and heaviness in the chest.

EMOTIONAL PATTERNS

Joy, over-excitement, sadness, excessive laughing, or crying, lack of emotions, bad manners, abusive nature, anger, nausea, dizziness, easily upset, type A personality, compulsive behaviors, insecurity, hostility, guilt, timid, does not like to make friends, does not trust anyone.

RELATED MUSCLES

Subscapularis, abdominalis, supra spinatus.

RELATED TIME: 11 a.m. - 1 a.m.

DENTAL CONNECTION

Subscapularis associated with upper lateral incisors.

ESSENTIAL NUTRITION

Calcium, vitamin C, vitamin E, and B complex.

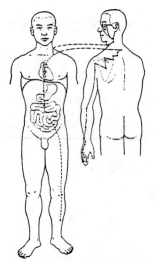

Figure 9-6.   Small Intestine Channel

SMALL INTESTINE CHANNEL

This channel originates at the ulnar side of the tip of the little finger and ascends along the ulnar side of the hand to the wrist emerging at the styloid process of the ulna. From here it travels directly upward along the posterior aspect of the ulna, passing between the olecranon of the ulna and the medial epicondyle of the humerus at the medical side of the elbow. It then proceeds along the posterior border of the lateral aspect of the upper arm, emerging behind the shoulder joint and circling around the superior and inferior fossa of the scapula. At the top of the shoulder, it crosses the bladder channel at acupuncture joints B 36 (Fufen) and B 11 (Dazhu), and the governing channel at acupuncture point Gv 14 (Dazhu), where the channel turns downward into the supraclavicular fossa, and connects with the heart. From here it descends along the esophagus and crosses the diaphragm to the stomach. Before reaching its associated organ, the small intestine, the channel intersects the conception channel internally and very deep, at acupuncture points Co 13 (Shangwan) and Co 12 (Zhongwan).

A branch of this channel travels upward from the supraclavicular fossa and crosses the neck and cheek to the outer canthus of the eye, where it meets the gall bladder channel at acupuncture point GB 1 (Tongziliao). Then it turns back across the temple and enters the ear at the small intestine acupuncture point SI 19 (Tinggong).

Another branch separates from the former branch on the cheek, ascends to the infraorbital region of the eye and then to the inner canthus, where it meets the bladder channel at acupuncture point B1. It then crosses horizontally to the zygomatic region.

Another branch descends to stomach acupuncture point St 39 (Xiajuxu), the lower uniting joint of the small intestine. This channel is associated with the small intestine and connects with the heart. It is also joined directly with the stomach.

Symptoms associated with the external course of this channel include numbness of the mouth and tongue, pain in the neck or cheek, sore throat, stiff neck, pain along the lateral aspect of the shoulder and upper arm.

Symptoms associated with the internal organ (small intestine) include pain and distension in the lower abdomen, possibly extending around the waist or to the genitals, diarrhea, abdominal pain with dry stool or constipation.

OVERACTIVE AND UNDERACTIVE MERIDIAN

The overactive meridian gives noisy intestinal movements, pain in the neck, and back of the shoulders. The underactive meridian causes odorless intestinal gas, unilateral headaches, pain around ears and under the cheek bone.

ACUTE ALLERGIC SYMPTOMS

Numbness of the mouth and tongue, pain in the neck, sore throat, stiff neck, pain along the channel, and lateral aspect of the shoulder and arm.

CHRONIC ALLERGIC SYMPTOMS

Pain, knee pain, shoulder pain, frozen shoulder, distention of lower abdomen, pain radiating around the waist and genitals, diarrhea, abdominal pain, with dry stool, or constipation.

EMOTIONAL PATTERNS

Joy, over excitement, absent mindedness, insecurity, feeling of abandonment or desertion, emotional instability, poor concentration, paranoia, day dreaming, sadness, sorrow, sighing, irritability, and easily annoyed, lacking the confidence to assert oneself, feeling shy, suppressing deep sorrow, becoming too involved with details, having a tendency to be introverted and easily hurt.

RELATED MUSCLES

Quadriceps, rectus abdominalis, and transverse abdominalis.

RELATED TIME: 1 - 3 p.m.

DENTAL CONNECTION

The quadriceps are associated with the first lower molar and rectus abdominalis are associated with the upper first molar.

ESSENTIAL NUTRITION

Vitamin B complex, vitamin D, vitamin E, acidophilus, yogurt, fibers, wheat germs, whole grains.

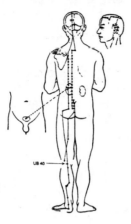

Figure 9-7.   Bladder Channel

BLADDER CHANNEL

This channel begins at the bladder channel acupuncture point B 1 (Jingming) at the inner canthus of the eye and ascends across the forehead, intersecting the governing channel at acupuncture point Gv 24 (Shenting), and the gall bladder channel at acupuncture point GB 20 (Baihui).

From here a branch descends to the area above the ear joining the gall bladder channel at acupuncture points GB 7 (Qubin), GB 8 (Shuaigu), Gb 12 (Wangu), etc.

A vertical branch enters the brain at the vertex and intersects with the governing channel at point Gv 17 (Naohu), before emerging and descending along nape of the neck and the muscles of the medial aspect of the scapula. Here the bladder channel meets the governing channel at acupuncture points Gv 14

(Dazhui) and Gv 13 (Taodao), after which it continues downward parallel to the spine, to the lumbar region. The channel then enters the internal cavity via the paravertebral muscles, communicating with the kidneys, and finally joins its associated organ, the bladder. Another branch separates in the lumbar region, crosses the buttock, and descends to the popliteal fossa of the knee.

Yet another branch separates from the main channel at the back of the neck and descends parallel to the spine, from the medial side of the scapula to the gluteal region. Here it crosses the buttock to intersect the gall bladder channel at acupuncture point GB 30 (Huantiao), and then descends across the lateral posterior aspect of the thigh to join with the other branch of this channel in the popliteal fossa continuing downward through the gastrocnemius muscle. The channel emerges behind the external malleolus, then follows the fifth metatarsal bone crossing its tuberosity to the lateral lip of the little toe at bladder acupuncture point B 67 (Zhiyin).

The bladder channel connects behind the knee with its lower uniting acupuncture point B 54 (Weizhong). This channel is associated with the bladder and connects with the kidneys. It is also joined directly with the brain and heart.

Symptoms associated with the external pathway of this channel include alternating chills and fever, headache, stiff neck, pain in the lumbar region, nasal congestion, disease of the eye, pain along the back of the leg and foot and pain along the meridians.

Symptoms associated with the internal organs (bladder) include pain in the lower abdomen, enuresis, retention of urine, painful urination, mental disorders.

OVERACTIVE AND UNDERACTIVE MERIDIAN

The overactive state causes one to have nagging low back ache with radiculitis (sciatic neuralgia to the legs). The underactive state causes upper and middle back ache, frequent urination, bed wetting in children or incontinence of urine.

ACUTE ALLERGIC SYMPTOMS

Frequent urination, painful or burning urination, loss of bladder control, bloody urine, chills, fever, headaches especially at the back of the neck, stiff neck, pain in the lower back, nasal congestion, disease of the eye, pain along back of the leg and foot, pain along the meridian, sciatic neuralgia, spasms of the calf muscles, pain in the lateral part of the ankle, pain in the lateral part of the sole, pain in the little toe, weakness in the rectum and rectal muscle, pain behind the knee, spasm behind the knee, and pain and discomfort in the lower abdomen.

CHRONIC ALLERGIC SYMPTOMS

Pain in the lower abdomen, enuresis, retention of urine, painful urination, mental disorders, pain in the fingers and toes, arthritis of the joints of little finger and to pain and stiffness of the back, chronic headaches at the back of the neck, pain in the inner canthus of the eyes, pain behind the knees, sciatic neuralgia, pain, muscle wasting, spasms, along the posterior part of the thigh, and leg along the meridian.

EMOTIONAL PATTERN

Timid, inefficient, annoyed, highly irritable, fearful unhappy, restless, impatience, and frustrated.

RELATED MUSCLES

Peroneus, sacrospinalis, anterior tibial, and posterior tibial.

RELATED TIME: 3 - 5 PM

DENTAL CONNECTION

2nd lower molar

ASSOCIATED NUTRITION

Vitamin C, A, E, B complex, B1, calcium, trace minerals.

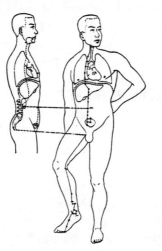

Figure 9-8. Kidney Channel

KIDNEY CHANNEL

This channel begins beneath the little toe, across the sole of the foot and emerges at kidney acupuncture point K 2 (Rangu) on the inferior aspect of the navicular tuberosity at the instep. From here it travels posterior to the medial malleolus, enters the heel, and proceeds upward along the medial aspect of the lower leg, where it intersects the spleen channel at acupuncture point Sp 6 (Sanyinjiao). Continuing up the leg within the gastrocnemius muscle, the channel traverses the medial aspect of the popliteal fossa and the medial, posterior aspect of the thigh to the base of the spine, where it intersects the governing channel at acupuncture point Gv 1 (Changqiang). Here it threads its way beneath the spine to enter its associated organ, the kidney, and to communicate with the bladder. It intersects the conception channel at acupuncture points Co 4 (Guanyuan) and Co 3 (Zongji).

A branch ascends directly from the kidney, across the liver and diaphragm, enters the lung, and follows the throat to the root of the tongue.

Another branch separates in the lung, connects with the heart, and disperses in the chest.

This channel is associated with the kidneys and connects with the bladder. It is also joined directly with the liver, lungs, heart and other organs.

Symptoms associated with the external pathways of the channel include pain along the lower vertebrae, low back pain, coldness in the feet, motor impairment or muscular atrophy of the foot, dryness of the mouth, sore throat, pain in the sole of the foot or along the posterior aspect of the leg or thigh, and pain along the meridians.

Symptoms related to the internal organ (kidney) include vertigo, facial edema, blurred vision, irritability, loose stools, chronic diarrhea or constipation, abdominal distension, vomiting and impotence.

OVERACTIVE AND UNDERACTIVE MERIDIAN

The overactive state gives high energy, high stamina, high immune system, good appetite and high fertility. The underactive state causes one to be timid, lack courage, lack self-assurance, lack sexual interest and have low fertility.

ACUTE ALLERGIC SYMPTOMS

Pain in the lower back, coldness in the back, coldness in the feet, spasms of the ankle and the feet, pain in the course of the channel, swelling in the legs, puffy eyes, bags under the eyes, dark circles under the eyes, motor impairment or muscular atrophy of the foot, dryness of the mouth, sore throat, pain in the sole of the foot, pain in the posterior aspect of the leg or thigh, ringing in the ears, pain in the ears, nagging mild asthma, tiredness, excessive sleeping, excessive salivation, nausea, light headedness, frequent urination, and burning or painful urination.

CHRONIC ALLERGIC SYMPTOMS

Vertigo, facial edema, blurred vision, irritability, loose stools, chronic diarrhea, constipation, abdominal distention, vomiting, tiredness, ringing in the ears, swollen ankles, fever, fever with chills, dry mouth, excessive thirst, poor appetite, poor memory, lack of concentration, and impotence.

EMOTIONAL PATTERNS

Indecision, fear, caution, seek attention, unable to express feelings.

RELATED MUSCLES

Psoas, upper trapezius, iliacus.

RELATED TIME: 5 - 7 p.m.

DENTAL CONNECTION

The Psoas muscle is associated with the lower 3rd molar.

ASSOCIATED NUTRITION

Vitamin A, E, B, essential fatty acids, calcium, and iron.

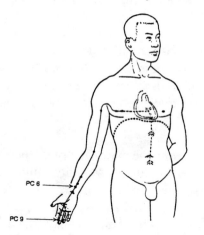

Figure 9-9. Pericardium Channel

PERICARDIUM CHANNEL

This channel begins in the chest where it joins its associated organ, the pericardium. It then descends across the diaphragm and into the abdomen, where it connects successively with the upper, middle, and lower warmers of the triple warmer organ.

A branch of the main channel runs along the chest emerging superficially in the costal region at pericardium channel acupuncture point 1, three units below the anterior axillary fold ascending to the inferior aspect of the axilla. From here it descends along the medial aspect of the upper arm between the paths of the lung and heart channels to the antecubital fossa, and then proceeds down the forearm between the tendons of palmaris longus and flexor carpi radialis muscles. Entering the palm, it follows the ulnar aspect of the middle finger until it reaches the finger tip.

Another branch separates in the palm and proceeds along the lateral aspect of the fourth finger of the fingertip. This channel is associated with the pericardium and is connected with the triple warmer organ.

Symptoms associated with the external course of this channel include stiff neck, spasms in the arm or leg, flushed face, pain in the eyes, sub-axillary swelling, spasms and contracture of the elbow and arm, restricting movements, hot palms, and pain along the channel.

Symptoms associated with the internal organ (pericardium) include impaired speech, fainting, irritability, fullness in the chest, heaviness in the chest mainly in the left side, motor impairment of the tongue, palpitations, chest pain, mental disorders, heaviness of the chest due to extreme emotional changes.

OVERACTIVE AND UNDERACTIVE MERIDIAN

The overactive state causes one to have dull headaches, heaviness in the head, upper abdominal distress and dream disturbed sleep.

The underactive state causes one to have various phobias like fear of heights (agoraphobia), fear of crowds, fear of closed areas (claustrophobia), insomnia, somnambulism (sleep walking), continuous chain of thoughts, and mental restlessness.

ACUTE ALLERGIC SYMPTOMS

Impaired speech, stiff neck, spasms in the arm, spasms in the leg, fainting spells, flushed face, irritability, fullness in the chest, heaviness in the chest, slurred speech, sensation of hot or cold, nausea, nervousness, pain in the eyes, submaxillary swellings, spasms of the elbow and arm, frozen shoulder, restricting movements, hot palms, and pain along the channels.

CHRONIC ALLERGIC SYMPTOMS

Contractures of the arm, or elbow, irritability, excessive appetite, fullness in the chest, sugar imbalance, sciatic neuralgia, pain in the anterior part of the thigh, pain in the medial part of the knee, the motor impairment of the tongue, palpitation, chest pain, and heaviness in the chest due to emotional overload.

EMOTIONAL PATTERNS

Joy, over excitement, regret, jealousy, sexual tension, stubbornness, manic disorders, heaviness in the head, light sleep with dreams, fear of heights, various phobias, imbalance in the sexual energy like never having enough sex, or in some cases no sexual desire.

RELATED MUSCLES

Gluteus medius, adductors, piriformis, gluteus maximus.

RELATED TIME: 7 - 9 p.m.

DENTAL CONNECTION

The gluteus maximus muscles are associated with lower cuspid, the gluteus medius are associated with lower central incisors and the piriformis and adductors are associated with lower lateral incisors.

ESSENTIAL NUTRITION

Vitamin E, vitamin C, chromium, and trace minerals.

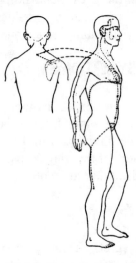

Figure 9-10.   Triple Burner Channel

TRIPLE WARMER CHANNEL

This channel is also referred to as triple burner channel or San Jiao channel. The triple warmer channel originates on the ulnar aspect of the fourth fingertip, ascends between the fourth and fifth metacarpal bones on the dorsum of the wrist, traverses the forearm between the ulna and radius and continues upward across the olecranon and the lateral aspect of the upper arm to the shoulder. It then intersects the small intestine channel at acupuncture point SI 12 (Bingfeng) and meets the governing channel at point GV 14 (Dazhui) before crossing back over the shoulder. It then intersects the gall bladder channel at acupuncture point GB 21 (Jianjing), from which it enters the supraclavicular fossa and travels to the mid chest region at conception channel point Co 17 (Shanzhong) and ascends to emerge superficially from the supraclavicular fossa at the neck. Here it proceeds upward behind the ear, intersecting the gall bladder channel at points GB 6 (Xuanli) and GB 4 (Hanyan) on the forehead before winding downward across the cheek to below the eye. It intersects the small intestine channel at point SI 18 (Quanliao).

Another branch separates behind the auricle and enters the ear. It then emerges in front of the ear, where it intersects the small intestine channel at point SI 19 (Tinggong), crosses in front of the gall bladder channel at point GB 3 (Shangguan) and traverses the cheek to terminate at the outer canthus at gall bladder channel point GB 23 (Sizhukong).

The triple warmer channel connects with its lower uniting bladder channel point B 53 (Weiyang). This branch of the triple warmer channel emerges from bladder point B 53 (Weiyang) and follows the course of the bladder channel to join with the bladder. This channel is associated with the triple warmer and is connected with the pericardium.

Symptoms associated with the external course of this channel include swelling and pain in the throat, pain in the cheek and jaw, redness in the eyes, deafness, pain behind the ear or along the lateral aspect of the shoulder and upper arm, and pain along the channel.

Symptoms associated with the internal organ (triple warmer) include abdominal distension, hardness and fullness in the lower abdomen, enuresis, frequent urination, edema, dysuria, excessive thirst, excessive hunger, and vertigo.

OVERACTIVE AND UNDERACTIVE MERIDIAN

The overactive state causes loss of hearing, ringing in the ears, tingling on the lateral part of the forearm and heavy or tight feeling in the elbow. The underactive meridian causes feeling of cold all over, tip of the fingers and toes become too cold and even may turn blue (Raynaud's syndrome).

ACUTE ALLERGIC SYMPTOMS

Swelling and pain in the throat, pain in the cheek and jaw, excessive hunger, redness in the eye, deafness, pain behind the ear, pain along the lateral aspect of the shoulder and upper arm, and pain along the channel.

CHRONIC ALLERGIC SYMPTOMS

Abdominal pain, distention, hardness and fullness in the lower abdomen, enuresis, frequent urination, edema, dysuria, excessive thirst, excessive hunger, always feels hungry even after eating a full stomach, vertigo, indigestion, constipation, pain in the medial part of the knee, shoulder pain, and fever in the late evening.

EMOTIONAL PATTERNS

Depression, despair, hopelessness, grief, excessive emotion, emptiness, deprivation, and phobias.

RELATED MUSCLES

Teres minor, sartorius, gracilis, soleus, and gastrocnemius,

RELATED TIME: 9 - 11 p.m.

DENTAL CONNECTIONS

The sartorius and the gracilis are associated with lower 1st molar.

ASSOCIATED NUTRITION

Iodine, trace minerals, vitamin C, Calcium, fluoride, and water.

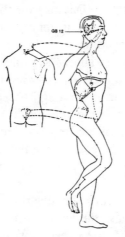

Figure 9-11.   Gall Bladder Channel

THE GALL BLADDER CHANNEL

This channel begins at the outer canthus of the eye and traverses the temple to the gall bladder channel point GB 22 (Heliao). It then ascends to the corner of the forehead where it intersects the stomach point S 8 (Touwei) before descending behind the ear. From here it proceeds along the neck in front of the triple warmer channel, crosses the small intestine channel at point SI 17 (Tianrong), then at the top of the shoulder, turns back and runs behind the triple warmer channel to intersect the governing channel at point GV 14 (Dazhui) on the spine. Finally the channel turns downward into the supraclavicular fossa.

One branch of the main channel emerges behind the auricle and enters the ear at gall bladder point GB 17 (Yifeng), emerging in front of the ear, this branch intersects the small intestine channel at SI 19 (Tinggong) and the stomach channel at S 7 (Xianguan) before terminating behind the outer canthus.

Another branch separates at the outer canthus and proceeds downward to stomach point S 5 (Daying) on the jaw. Then crossing the triple warmer channel it returns upward to the infraorbital region before descending again to the neck, where it joins the original channel in the supraclavicular fossa. From here it descends further into the chest, crossing the diaphragm and connecting with the liver before joining its associated organ, the gall bladder. Continuing along the inside of the ribs, it emerges in the inguinal region of the lower abdomen and winds around the genitals submerging again in the hip at gall bladder point GB 30(Huantiao).

Yet another vertical branch runs downward from the supraclavicular fossa to the axilla and the lateral aspect of the chest. It crosses the ribs and intersects the liver channel at point Lv 13 (Zhangmen) before turning back to the sacral region, where it crosses the bladder channel points B31 (Hangliao) to B 34 (Xialiao). This branch then descends to the hip joint, and continues down the lateral side of the thigh and knee, passing along the anterior aspect of the fibula to its lower end. Here it crosses in front of the lateral malleolus and traverses the dorsum of the foot, entering the same between the fourth and fifth metatarsal bones before terminating at the lateral side of the tip of the fourth toe, or gall bladder point GB 44 (Zugiaoyin).

Finally a branch separates on the dorsum of the foot at gall bladder point GB 41 (Zulinqi) and runs between the first and second metatarsal bones to the medial tip of the big toe, then crosses under the toenail to join with the liver channel at point Liv 1 (Dadun).

This channel connects with its lower uniting point gall bladder point GB 34 (Yanglingquan). It is associated with the gall bladder and connects with the liver. It is also joined directly with the heart.

Symptoms associated with the external course of this channel include alternating fever and chills, headache, ashen complexion, pain in the eye or jaw, swelling in subaxillary region, scrofula, deafness, pain along the channel in the hip region, leg or foot, and pain along the channel, tremors or twitching of the body or parts of the body.

Symptoms associated with the internal organ (gall bladder) include pain in the ribs, vomiting, bitter taste in the mouth, and chest pain, moving pains in the joints.

OVERACTIVE AND UNDERACTIVE MERIDIAN

The overactive state causes a feeling of heaviness in the head and upper abdomen, pain in the upper abdomen and pain and cramps along the anterolateral abdominal wall. The underactive state causes one to be in a acidosis condition, which causes a person to sigh, feel cold, have dizzy spells, light headedness, and a tendency to be sloppy and stumble.

ACUTE ALLERGIC SYMPTOMS

Alternating fever and chills, headaches, ashen complexion, pain in the eye, pain in the jaw, swelling in the submaxillary region, scrofula, deafness, pain along the gall bladder channel, pain in the hip, leg foot, a heavy sensation in the right upper part of the abdomen, tremors, twitching, pain and cramps along the anterolateral wall, sighing, dizziness, chills, fever, yellowish complexion.

CHRONIC ALLERGIC SYMPTOMS

Pain in the intercostal areas, vomiting, bitter taste in the mouth, chest pain, moving arthritis, pain in the right side of the abdomen, pain along the channel, problem to digest fats, nausea with fried foods.

EMOTIONAL PATTERN

Rage, assertion, aggression, shouting, and talking aloud.

RELATED MUSCLE Anterior deltoid and popliteus.

RELATED TIME: 11 p.m. - 1 a.m.

DENTAL CONNECTION The popliteus is associated with the upper first bicuspid and the deltoid is associated with upper cuspid.

ESSENTIAL NUTRITION Vitamin A, calcium, linoleic acids and oleic acids.

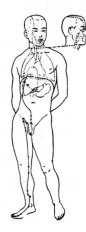

Figure 9-12. Liver Channel

LIVER CHANNEL

This channel begins on the dorsum of the big toe, continues across the foot to a point one unit in front of the medial malleolus and proceeds upward to Spleen channel acupuncture point Sp 6 (sanyinjiao) where it intersects the spleen channel. From here it continues to the medial aspect of the lower leg, recrossing the spleen channel eight units above the medial malleolus, and there after running posterior to that channel over the knee and thigh. Winding around the genitals, the channel enters the lower abdomen where it meets the conception channel at points CO 2 (Qugu), Co 3 (Zhongji) and Co 4 (Guanyuan) before skirting the stomach and joining with its associated organ, the liver, and connecting with the gall bladder. Then the channel continues upward, across the diaphragm and costal region, traverses the nasopharynx, connecting with the tissue surrounding the eye. Finally, the channel ascends across the forehead and meets the governing channel at the vertex.

A branch separates below the eye and encircles the inside of the lips.

Another branch separates in the liver, crosses the diaphragm and reaches the lung. This channel is associated with the liver and connects with the gall bladder. It is also joined directly with the lungs, stomach, kidneys, brain and other organs.

Symptoms associated with the external courses of the channel include headaches, vertigo, blurred vision, tinnitus, fever, spasms in the extremities, pain along the channel.

Symptoms associated with the internal organ (liver) include fullness or pain in the costal region or chest, hard lumps in the upper abdomen, abdominal pain, vomiting, jaundice, loose stool, pain in the lower abdomen, hernia, enuresis, retention of the urine, dark urine, dizziness, stoke like conditions, irregular menses, pre-menstrual syndromes, reproductive organ disturbances, excessive bright-colored bleeding during menses.

OVERACTIVE AND UNDERACTIVE MERIDIAN

A person with an overactive meridian is very excitable and cries easily. He or she would start on several different projects at once and goes in different directions at one time. But he or she may have an obsession to keep going until everything is done.

ACUTE ALLERGIC SYMPTOMS

Headache is at the top of the head, vertigo, blurred vision, feeling of some obstruction in the throat, tinnitus, fever, spasms in the extremities and pain along the channel.

CHRONIC ALLERGIC SYMPTOM

Pain in the intercostal region, PMS, pain in the breasts, hard lumps in the upper abdomen, abdominal pain, vomiting, jaundice, loose stools, pain in the lower abdomen, hernia, enuresis, retention of urine, dark urine, dizziness, stroke like condition, irregular menses, PMS, reproductive organ disturbances, excessive bright colored bleeding during menses.

EMOTIONAL PATTERNS

Anger, aggression, unhappiness, complaining all the time, and finding faults with others.

RELATED TIME: 1 - 3 a.m.

RELATED MUSCLE

Pectoralis major sternal, rhomboideus.

DENTAL CONNECTION

The pectoralis major sternal muscle is associated with the lower second bicuspid.

ESSENTIAL NUTRITION

Beets, green vegetables, vitamin A, trace minerals and unsaturated fatty acids.

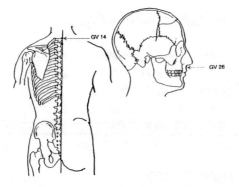

Figure 9-13. Governing Vessel Channel
GOVERNING VESSEL

This channel is the confluence of all the yang channels, over which is said to "govern." There are four paths followed by the channel. This first originates in the perineum and ascends along the middle of the spine, until it reaches point Gv 16 (Fengfu) at the nape of the neck. Here it enters the brain, ascends to the vertex, and follows the midline of the forehead across the bridge of the nose, terminating at the upper lip.

The second path begins in the pelvic region, descends to the genitals and perineum, then passes through the tip of the coccyx. Here it diverts into the gluteal region where it intersects the kidney and bladder channels before returning to the spinal column and then joining with the kidneys.

The origin of the third path is in common with that of the bladder channel at the inner canthus of the eye. The two (bilateral) branches, from each of the inner canthi, ascend across the forehead and converge at the vertex where the channel enters the brain. Emerging at the lower end of the nape of the neck, the channel again divides into two branches which descend along the opposite sides of the spine to the waist. Here they join with the kidneys.

Finally, the fourth path of the governing channel begins in the lower abdomen and rises directly across the navel, passes through the heart and enters the trachea. Continuing its upward course, the channel crosses the cheek and encircles the mouth, before terminating at a point below the middle of the eye.

This channel intersects the bladder channel at point B 12 (Fengmen), and the conception channel at point Co 1 (Iluiyin).

Pathological symptoms: because this channel supplies the brain and spinal region and intersects the liver channel at the vertex, obstruction of its qi may result in symptoms such as stiffness and pain along the spinal column. Deficient qi in the channel may produce a heavy sensation in the head, vertigo and shaking. Mental disorders may be attributed to wind entering the brain through this channel. Febrile diseases are commonly associated with the governing channel, and, because one branch of the channel ascends through the abdomen, when the channel is unbalanced, its qi rushes upward toward the heart. Symptoms such as colic, constipation, enuresis, hemorrhoids and functional infertility may result.

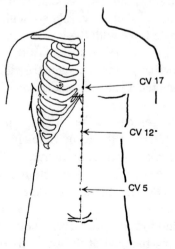

Figure 9-14. Conception Vessel Channel

CONCEPTION VESSEL CHANNEL

This channel has two routes. The first arises in the lower abdomen below conception vessel acupuncture point Cv 3 (Zhongji), ascends along the midline of the abdomen and chest, across the throat and jaw, and finally winds around the mouth, terminating in the region of the eye.

The second course arises in the pelvic cavity, enters the spine and ascends along the back.

This channel intersects the stomach channel at acupuncture point stomach 1 (Chenqi) and the governing vessel at the acupuncture point Gv 28 (Yinjiao).

PATHOLOGICAL SYMPTOMS

The conception vessel channel is the confluence of the Yin channels. Therefore, abnormality along the conception channel will appear principally in pathological symptoms of the Yin channels, especially symptoms associated with the liver and kidneys. Its function is closely related with pregnancy and, therefore has intimate links with the kidneys and uterus. If its qi is deficient, infertility or other disorders of the urogenital system may result. Leukorrhea, irregular menstruation, colic, etc., are all symptoms associated with the conception channel.

Any possible allergen can cause blockage in one meridian or more than one meridians at the same time. If it is blocking only one meridian, the patient may demonstrate symptoms related to that particular blocked meridian. The intensity of the symptoms will depend on the severity of the blockage. Again, the patient may suffer from one symptom, many symptoms or all the symptoms of the said blocked meridian. Sometimes patients can have many meridians blocked at the same time. In such cases, the patient may demonstrate varieties of symptoms, one from each meridian or many from some meridians and one or two from others. Some patients with just one meridian block can demonstrate one symptom only but with great intensity. In some people, even though all the meridians are blocked, the patient may not show much reaction at all. These variations with all these possibilities make the diagnosis difficult in some cases.

CHAPTER TEN

MORE ON NAMBUDRIPAD'S TECHNIQUES OF ALLERGY ELIMINATION

Most of the acupuncture points used to eliminate energy blockages lie near some vital organs. The information about the treatment points and techniques for needling the specific points to remove allergy are not described in this book. Each of these points are needled with special techniques which are taught in acupuncture colleges. Teaching these techniques is beyond the scope of this book and is purposely excluded. Needling in these areas requires proper education and much practice. Improper needling can cause damage to the vital organs and cause greater damage to health, sometimes causing fatal accidents and even death. There are hundreds of doctors trained in NAET treatment methods all over the country. If you can not find one near you, please refer to the telephone number on the back of the book for information.

Information about few important acupuncture points are given in this chapter. They can be used to help to get control of any mild to moderate allergic reactions. Severely allergic patients should consult a licensed acupuncturist for treatments. Stimulation of these points will not remove the allergies. This will help to remove the energy blockages temporarily.

We have seen the common routes of the meridians, their internal pathways and external routes (diagrams 9-1 to 9-12). We have also seen how these meridians get blocked from simple allergies and give rise to specific pathological, physical, physiological, and emotional symptoms in the body. In Chapter 6, "Muscle-Response testing for Allergy," we learned to test for allergies. Allergies may be the causative agent for energy blockages in particular meridians. We have learned to test for allergies in general. The reader is urged to practice these testing techniques and make a habit of testing everything before one uses food, cloths, make-up, chemicals, etc.

ISOLATING THE BLOCKAGES

Testing and isolating the particular blockages can be done in many ways. One of the methods is described here and it is fairly easy to understand and can be learned by anyone with some practice.

STEP 1 Balance the patient and find an indicator muscle. Refer to Chapter 6, "Muscle-Response Testing for Allergies" for details.

STEP 2 Patient lies down on his back with the allergen (e.g., an apple) in his resting palm. (Surrogate testing can also be used when it is needed.)

STEP 3 Tester touches the points in diagram 10-1, one at a time, and tests the indicator muscles. For example, touch point "1" in diagram 10.1 with the finger tips of one hand and with the other hand test the indicator muscle, while the patient is still holding the allergen in his one hand. The muscle goes weak. This indicates that the meridian, or the energy pathways connected to that particular point, has energy blockages.

Point "1" relates to the lung channel. Obstruction in the free flow of energy can be anywhere in the lung channel. Test the indicator muscle, while touching each point in the lung channel (for more information regarding point location in the channels refer to the appropriate books on acupuncture given in the bibliography). The indicator muscle gets weakest when the tester touches sites of the blocked area in the meridian. For point-meridian relationships refer to table 10-1. This way one can trace all the weak meridians and specific weak sites in one's body.

Table 10-1

Point Name	No. Related Meridians
Pt 1	Lu 1 Lung
Pt 2	Cv 17 Pericardium
Pt 3	Liv 14 Liver
Pt 4	GB 24 Gall bladder
Pt 5	CV 14 Heart
Pt 6	CV 12 Stomach
Pt 7	GB 25 Kidney
Pt 8	Liv 13 Spleen
Pt 9	St25 Large Intestine
Pt 10	CV5 Tri-Heater
Pt 11	CV4 Small Intestine
Pt 12	CV3 Bladder

Finger pressure therapy can be used to restore the energy flow temporarily in the blocked energy meridians.

STEP 1 The first step for finger pressure therapy is to find the organ or meridian that is being blocked. Find the related organ point.

Table 10-1

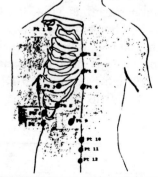

STEP 2   Apply slight finger pressure with the pad of your index finger on the point.   Hold 60 seconds at each point. Follow the order of the sequence of the points given in the previous page. When the blocked organ is found, make that as a starting point to do the energy balancing. For example, if the energy is blocked in the liver meridian, make the liver organ point the first point to start the finger pressure. If the heart is found to be blocked, use the heart point as the first point in the sequence of energy balancing.

STEP 3   Hold 60 seconds at each point and go through all 12 points and come back to the starting point.   Then hold 60 seconds at the starting point and stop the treatment. Always end at the starting point, this completes the energy cycle.

Some patients can experience physical or emotional pain or emotional release during these treatment sessions. If the patient has an emotional blockage, it needs to be isolated and treated to the maximum result. Some patients can get tingling pains, sharp pains, pulsations, excessive perspiration, etc. during the treatment. In such instances, please go through another cycle of treatment. Sometimes this can solve the problem.

Some commonly used acupuncture points and their uses to help in emergency situations are given below. Massage these points gently with the finger pads for one minute each. Please refer to the appropriate meridians in chapter 9 to find the location of these points.

1. Fainting: Gv 26, GB 12, LI 1, Pc 9

2. Nausea: CV 12, Pc 6

3. Backache: Gv 26, UB 40

4. Fatigue: CV 5, LI 1, CV17

5. Fever: LI 11, LU 10, GV14

For more information on revival techniques, refer to Chapter 3, pages 570 to 573, in Acupuncture: A Comprehensive Text, by Shanghai College of Traditional Medicine, Eastland Press, 1981.

A WORD TO THE ALLERGIC PATIENT

The author has tried to discuss most of the various types of allergic manifestations, more common types of allergic reactions, and prevalent Western and Oriental methods of treatments of allergies.   She has presented enough information on Nambudripad's Allergy Elimination Treatment, which could render the patient completely allergy-free from the allergens that have been already treated. She has also explained in detail how to test and find your allergies on your own, the most reliable method of allergy testing. This itself should help allergic patients control their allergies and prevent unexpected and unfortunate incidences by carefully preventing known allergens. It is hoped that the reader will spend some time in reading every page carefully and learning about this new discovery and many exciting case studies. Thousands of people have undergone these treatments already as examples have shown in these pages, and they now enjoy good health. Allergic patients do not have to spend the rest of their lives in fear or in a bubble anymore but can live like any other normal person, if they will get treated for their allergies by doctors trained in Nambudripad's Allergy Elimination Treatments.

It is hoped that the reader will take enough time to understand the material presented in this book; to learn about muscle response testing to find allergies, and to make use of the balancing techniques described here and the emergency measures

180

to pull them out of serious emergency situations by using Oriental medical techniques. Nambudripad's Allergy Elimination Techniques allergy specialists (acupuncturists, chiropractors, and allopathic medical; doctors with special training in Nambudripad's Allergy Elimination Techniques) are available at various locations in the country. Throughout the book, the author has attempted to emphasize the importance of full and complete cooperation between patient and allergist, for it is only by such complete cooperation that the best results can be obtained.

It is not sufficient for the patient to receive treatments regularly, although this is vitally important. He must also follow the other instructions if he hopes to attain the maximum result in a minimum of time. Allergy treatments require repeated office visits in the beginning and, once all the known allergies are eliminated, the patient is trained to find his own allergies. He then has to see the doctor only if he finds any item that bothers him or for annual follow-ups. All allergies cannot be eliminated in one or two office visits. In some severe cases, it may take as many as three visits a week for one or two years' duration to make them achieve a condition close to normalcy, depending on the patient's immune system response.

There have been a few patients who had mild cases of allergies and completed the treatments in one two visits or in two to three months and were not seen again, except occasionally. On the average, many of the other patients have taken anywhere from an eight to twelve month period to achieve satisfactory results. Some extreme cases have taken from two and a half to three years to solve all their problems. Allergic patients should keep this time span in mind when they approach any NAET specialists. If they are discontinued before completion of all the necessary treatments, the results will be unsatisfactory and allergic symptoms are very likely to recur. This will tend to make the patient feel that the allergy itself is to blame. For this reason, it is better not even to start treatment than to start and discontinue too soon, or to start and then cooperate in a half-hearted manner. The allergist will discharge his patients with proper instructions just as soon as he feels it is safe to do so.

How can patients cooperate and help the doctor achieve maximum results in minimum time? After each treatment, patients are advised to stay away from the treated item for 24 hours. There are 12 energy meridians. In order for an energy molecule to pass through one meridian it takes two hours. To circulate through 12 meridians, it takes 24 hours. This means that the patient should not even come close to the object as its electromagnetic field can interfere with the patients own field and negate the treatment. Patients are also advised to maintain a food diary. Thus, if the patient reacts to something violently during treatment, the offender can be easily traced and treated thus preventing further pain. During treatment patients are placed on a strict diet of nonallergic items after completion of three treatments. This helps the body to maintain good health without having to face possible allergic items and speeds up the treatment process while reducing interference.

The following is a list of general directions which it is hoped will be of assistance to allergic patients regardless of the particular manifestations from which they may suffer.

1. The best time to begin treatment for your allergic symptoms is now. Do not wait until the next attack. It is not likely that the symptom will decrease with the passing of time; but more likely they will become more severe.

2. Report regularly for treatment and as often as directed by your allergy doctor. If necessary, long periods of breaks should be taken only after completion of each item. Never take more than two days off without completing treatment for each item. For example, when getting treated for a milk allergy, if one took five consecutive visits to clear the allergy, he should take a few

days or a week off from treatments. After being cleared of the milk and before starting treatment for another item like beef, one may take the vacation. If one exposes the brain to an allergen, but does not complete the treatment, unpleasant consequences or exaggeration of the problem can result.

Such was the case of a 28 year old woman who was treated for cotton. After seven consecutive treatments, she decided to go on a short vacation before being cleared of her allergy and without letting the allergist know. Three months later her husband called the allergist and asked whether she could help his wife's present condition. Two days into her vacation, she had slipped into a depression and refused to talk to or cooperate with anyone. (She had a nervous breakdown when she was a teenager and she had recovered from that episode completely.) Finally, the husband took her to a psychologist and therapist, neither of whom could help her come out of the depression. The allergist remembered that she had not completed treatment for cotton. She was brought into the office and treated for cotton and was cleared after four more treatments, a total of eleven. At the end of these treatments, she came out of her depression and became normal again. Here is a clear example of the danger of letting go of treatments in midstream.

3. Certain people may have a negative reaction to a treatment. One cannot predict reactions ahead of time. For this reason, the patient has to remain in the doctor's office anywhere from a half an hour to an hour following the treatment. During that time, if there is an unusual reaction, the doctor will treat the patient further. If there is no reaction, the patient will be sent home with certain instructions to be followed.

4. The patient is not supposed to come close to the energy field of the allergic items after he leaves the doctor's office for a period of 24 hours. This is a crucial time, because the brain works on a biological time clock of 24-hour cycles. During this time, the brain can reject or accept the treatment. If the brain accepts the treatment, then it will probably not reject it for the rest of the patient's life.

The brain's acceptance of the allergen as an ally will also make necessary changes in the chemical activity of the body and its functions. It is probable, and quite likely, that this is also capable of making changes in the genes, RNA, and DNA. We have not conducted experiments in the genetics field, but whenever a pregnant woman gets treated and clears an allergy her child does not react to the mother's allergen when it is born. When couples get treated for their allergies before they have children, their offspring do not react to these items at all. This tends to support the theory that the children's genes have become adjusted so as not to react.

A 22 year old woman who had two miscarriages came to our office, and we found her to be allergic to most of the foods she was eating. She was treated for most of the items. By then she got pregnant again and discontinued the treatment at that time. This time she carried full term and had a normal child. Then she returned again for the treatment for herself as well as for the child. When the child was examined, he was found not to be allergic to the items the mother had passed before she got pregnant. He was allergic to the items for which the mother was not as yet treated.

A young couple, both of whom manifested a number of allergic problems like migraines, dizzy spells, sinusitis, joint pains etc., were treated for all their known allergies. Then they had a child. We checked the child and found that the child was absolutely healthy with no known allergies at all.

Another couple, who were allergic to many items, were treated for all the foods, but did not get treated for any fabrics. When the child was born, she developed severe rashes all over the body and could not wear any clothes. The parents brought the child in for evaluation, and we found she was allergic to all the fabrics, but not to food items.

5. Soon after treatment, patients should avoid strenuous activity, exercises, heavy meals, etc., for at least three to four hours. It is possible that any of these activities can cause a sudden blockage in the energy pathway and thus cause unpleasant reactions.

6. Patients who are allergic to many items will experience various symptoms from using the allergenic items while they are getting treated. In this type of treatment, the patient is asked to use or eat anything he wants except for the item for which he is getting treated. If he is eating some other allergen, he can still react to that particular allergen even though this does not interfere with the ongoing treatment. The only exception is that the patient may not feel very good. For better and faster results, the patient should avoid all other allergens. If the patient is under any other medical care for any other symptoms, he is advised to continue those other treatments as before, along with the NAET treatments. This will help the patient keep his other health problems under control while going through the allergy treatment. Thus, the body does not have to fight stress or diseases from different causes at the same time as the stress of the new treatment. Patients who have asthma, migraine headaches, or other illnesses, when they continue their anti-asthma medicines or pain killers, can more easily get through these allergy treatments than patients who refuse to seek Western medical supportive treatments and rely on the allergy treatment alone.

7. Patients are advised to try not to become exposed to extreme weather like heat, cold, drafts, while getting treated. Patients with a lot of allergies cannot tolerate extreme weather conditions, because they may be allergic to the physical agents as explained before.

8. Patients are advised to practice good nutrition. They should try to eat nonallergenic items, or items for which they have already been treated, while going through this treatment program. Patients are also advised not to overeat or overexercise, to drink plenty of liquids, and get plenty of rest.

9. Remember, it usually takes several years to build up a sensitivity to the point where severe reactions occur. Do not get discouraged if relief from symptoms is delayed for some time. Just because all the symptoms do not disappear at the end of a few days' or weeks' treatment, there is no reason for discontinuing a diet or the treatments. When a few major allergies are cleared, minor allergies will be noticed more easily. Your awareness of allergies will be more pronounced after a few items have been cleared. Some patients ask, "After being cleared for some items, do I become more allergic to things I was not allergic to before?" The answer is a definite "No." The person's awareness increases, or the allergic reactions stick out more noticeably after some major items have been cleared.

For example, before treatment a patient was never told that he had allergies whenever he had a sore throat, headache, or body ache. He thought he had caught a "flu" or a virus, and probably ran to get some antibiotics. Whatever he may take, it will normally take 7 to 21 days to get better. Now whenever he gets a sore throat, etc., he will begin to search for the reason, "What did I eat that was different?" and will find the answer. "Oh! It was that piece of pineapple I ate in the fruit salad that is causing these flu like symptoms." So, actually your allergy does not increase, you just become more aware of its manifestations.

10. Avoid emotional stress and undue worry. This will bring down the immune system by increasing the energy blockages and cause more allergic reactions.

11. As you improve and your symptoms grow less severe and less frequent, do not stop the treatments. Try to complete treatments for all your known allergies. Otherwise, untreated allergies may build up and cause problems later.

12. Severely allergic patients should always try to carry antihistamines and oral medications or adrenalin shots with them. Severely allergic patients can get into life threatening situations at any time with any kind of allergies. If the patient can get the adrenalin shot or antihistamines immediately, the after-affect of the reaction will be less and any unfortunate incidents can be prevented.

Additional, specific instructions will be necessary for each patient and will vary depending on the patient's sensitivities and allergic manifestations. These instructions will be provided by the allergy specialist.

Statistics show that from 80 to 90 percent of allergic patients, who receive proper treatments by NAET treatments and cooperate with the doctor, are entirely relieved of any allergy related problems or are satisfactorily improved. With these odds in your favor and the proper confidence in your NAET allergist, you should stand a good chance of being among those who carry on a normal life and enjoy the good health you so greatly desire. Above all, do not get discouraged and try to give yourself enough time for your body to get well. Give it the second chance it deserves.

Allergy patients in the process of being treated are often under great stress. Many have weak immune systems. Most suffer from various allergy related illnesses that may affect the physical, psychological and/or physiological aspects of their health. The intensity and nature of the symptoms vary from patient to patient, depending on the effect on their blocked nerve supply (meridians or energy pathways) to the relevant part of the brain. Refer to Chapter 9 for discussion of the pathological functions of the acupuncture meridians.

When a patient is treated with NAET Techniques, the blocked meridians will be opened and energy will be released. Thus, the related organs and nerve pathways can function normally once again. Sometimes when more than one meridian is blocked, when the blockage is chronic in nature or when the immune system is lowered due to chronic illness, it is likely that such patients may need more treatments. If the allergy is not cleared in one treatment, the remaining blocked meridians can cause exaggerated symptoms until the patient has been treated and cleared of the allergy.

For example, a patient suffered blockage of the stomach and large intestine channels. When the blockage of the stomach channel is cleared, but the large intestine is not cleared the patient might experience severe constipation or any or all other symptoms related to the large intestine channel until the allergen is completely desensitized. When liver, kidney and stomach channels are affected and if the kidney channel is cleared with the first treatment and liver and stomach channels did not clear, then the patient will experience the pathological symptoms related to liver and stomach channels. Such a patient can experience severe mood swings, emotional instability, etc., related to the liver and severe migraines, nausea, indigestion, etc., related to the stomach channel. The kidney channel blockages could have resulted in severe back pains and tiredness prior to the treatment, but when the kidney channel cleared of the energy blockage with the first treatment, the patient could experience complete relief of the kidney channel related symptoms. The other symptoms will persist until all the meridians are cleared of the blockage.

Although the treatment may appear simple to the onlooker, the strain on the patient is considerable. To start with, rigidly avoiding any contact with the allergen demand certain sacrifices. Patients may have to deal with certain possible pathological symptoms in those cases where all the meridians have not assimilated the treatment. At this time, patients undergoing the treatment need all the support and understanding that family and friends can provide to put up with mood swings, shortness of temper, physical, physiological, and psychological disturbances, knowing that the patient will overcome these uncomfortable symptoms when the patient has successfully completed the treatment.

Some patients may use illness as a crutch and an excuse not to resume their former activities after the treatment. On the other hand, some employers consider people who have had severe allergies as problem employees, making it difficult to get back to work. Those who seek not to become involved in their former lifestyles should be guided to get into a different career of their interest. Family and friends should provide as much help and support through and after the treatment period to make the patient's life easier.

CHAPTER ELEVEN

ALLERGY AND THE RESPIRATORY SYSTEM

Hay fever has been recognized and diagnosed generally only recently as compared with other human ailments. Nevertheless, history records many instances of conditions which were undoubtedly hay fever, although not recognized as such. Even in time of Galen, the Greek physician who lived in the second century A.D., a record was made of persons who had an idiosyncrasy to roses. In the fourteenth century, according to one historian, the king of Poland had such a distaste for apples that he fled even from their aroma as if it were the most fatal poison. In 1563, Lusitanus described persons who suffered when smelling or eating cheese, as though it were poison. He also spoke of a friend who suffered attacks similar to hay fever at the mere sight of a rose. In 1693, it was said by Riedlin that the Duke of Schomberg could not bear the sight of a cat nor even the odor of a hidden one, without dizziness and difficulty in breathing. However, the work on hay fever, which became the foundation for our modern knowledge of this allergic disease, was done by John Bostock, an English physician.

In 1819, Dr. Bostock presented a paper before the medical society describing his own ailment, which he had seasonally since childhood. Nine years later, he published a paper covering his further studies of this subject, and called the condition "summer catarrh." In the meantime, however, it had come to be known as hay fever, the name which it still bears, in spite of the efforts of many physicians to change it.

The term hay fever is actually a misnomer and incorrectly describes this condition, as it seldom caused by hay, and only occasionally produces a fever. It may be defined as an allergic manifestation which occurs seasonally and is caused primarily by pollens, although it may be aggravated by other substances. It was called hay fever, because it was thought by many to be caused by hay; despite the fact that as early as 1831 John Elliotson, another English doctor, definitely stated that the condition was not caused by hay, but rather it had its origin in fresh flowers and grasses, and was probably due to pollens. For this reason, he had declared it should not be known by such a misleading name. Later research confirmed his opinion but the name has persisted and is still used by both doctors and the lay public to describe this particular allergic manifestation.

Allergic rhinitis (inflammation of the nose and nasal passages) causes symptoms which are very similar, are often present throughout the year, and are caused by other allergens, such as food, inhalants, fabrics or other substances. Because of the similarity in symptoms, allergic rhinitis is more perennial. Many patients suffer from both conditions at the same time, with the symptoms being considerably aggravated and increased during the pollen season.

Hay fever and allergic rhinitis are both characterized by symptoms of watery discharge from the nose, eyes, and throat, loss of taste and smell, and other symptoms similar to those accompanying colds. The three most common symptoms are severe sneezing, watery nasal discharge, and nasal obstruction, or stuffy nose. Many patients also complain of an annoying tickle inside the nose, which results in violent sneezing. Others have dry, hacking coughs, and some have a profuse watery secretion or discharge with practically no sneezing or obstruction of the nasal passages.

In children, it is very common for nasal blocking or stoppage of the nasal passages, to be the principal symptom. These children have a nasal twang to their voices and breathe through their mouths. If the condition is permitted to continue untreated it will frequently result in actual facial deformity in the children. Many patients, in addition to the above symptoms, complain of intense itching of the eyes, ears, throat, soft palate, and sometimes the face. In hay fever, the symptoms may vary considerably with various patients. Many hay fever patients are very sensitive to changes in temperature and weather, and their condition is usually aggravated by cool or damp air, although the pollen count is lower under these circumstances.

Most hay fever sufferers feel better in warm weather and when the sun is shining. This condition, like other allergic conditions, frequently causes the patient to have an almost constant feeling of chilliness, so that he requires more bedding and warmer clothing than persons not suffering from this ailment.

Many patients with hay fever, principally due to pollen allergy, will also be found to be allergic to certain foods, as well as other inhalants and contactants. The most common items seen causing hay fever, other than pollens and grasses, are sugar, carob, corn, wheat, beans, pineapple, tomato, banana, perfume, furniture, acts, dogs, feathers, kapok, dust, plastics, rubber and leather. Hay fever victims may often suffer from nasal polyps. These are swellings or growths of the mucus membrane which occur in the nostrils. They tend to become enlarged or shrunken, to some extent, as the other symptoms are aggravated or subside. They are due to congestion and inflammation of the mucus membrane which causes a swelling or overgrowth of these tissues. In some instances, they become large enough to completely block the nasal passages and even extend beyond the nostrils.

A 49-year-old patient had suffered nasal polyps (as well as other allergic manifestations including asthma), and had them removed several times by surgery. Since the operations did not in any sense correct the cause, they continued to return. Eventually, when she had reached the stage of being completely down and out, due to ill health and doctor bills, she heard about Nambudripad's treatment program through one of her childhood friends and visited our office. She was tested for various items, including pollens, trees, fabrics, chemicals and foods. Soon after beginning allergy treatments, polyps were removed again by surgery. She continued to receive allergy elimination treatments for a year following the surgery. Her general health improved, her asthma and other allergic symptoms got under control just by watching her diet and lifestyle. Nasal polyps also kept away for the past four years with out any sign of regrowth. The major progress in this treatment was made after she cleared the allergy for formaldehyde, which is seen in almost all the fabrics, wooden works, office products, paper works, inks, white-out, carpets and many household items.

It is extremely important that the hay fever patient consult an appropriate allergist with knowledge of Nambudripad's Allergy Elimination Treatment techniques as soon as possible after he realizes that he has this condition. As time goes by, it is very likely to become increasingly severe with each season, with the possibility of more serious complications with each severe hay fever attack. Also, if hay fever is allowed to continue untreated, the number of allergens to which the patient is sensitive is likely to increase, as well as the degree of sensitivity to the various allergens.

Allergic rhinitis may be caused by any substance, such as house dust, occupational dusts such as flour in the bakery, cosmetics, foods, household pets, animal danders, epitelials, chalk powder, newspaper ink, paint, plastics, chemical sprays, molds, soaps, perfumes and other chemical agents. The sooner proper treatment is begun in all types of allergies, the better it is for the patient. Prompt treatment also greatly lessens the likelihood that a comparatively mild allergic manifestation, such as hay fever or allergic rhinitis, will develop into a more severe allergy such as asthma.

Probably the most serious and disabling allergic condition from which sensitive individuals suffer is asthma. The word asthma comes from Greek meaning "I gasp for breath." It was used by

Hippocrates (460-370 B.C.) to denote certain types of breathing difficulties. This is an allergic state in which the bronchial tubes constrict the passage of air. This results in severe difficulty in breathing and a whistling type of exhalation (expelling the air from the lungs). Many times the patient also has a cough, which further aggravates his misery. These attacks occur spasmodically and are very severe at times. Often the sensation of suffocation is so great, in fact, that the patient feels he is choking to death and can not possibly last more than a few minutes longer. Sometimes, an attack of asthma does prove fatal and the patient dies from exhaustion and inability to breathe.

An allergic tendency toward asthma is inherited. As stated earlier, the tendency (although not the actual allergic disease) is inherited. It occurs much more frequently in families that have a history of various allergic conditions. However, in the case of asthma, the tendency toward this particular allergic ailment seems to be inherited more frequently than in most other allergic diseases. For instance, a woman who suffers from hay fever may have children who suffer from some other manifestations such as dermatitis, rather than hay fever, whereas a patient who suffers from asthma is quite likely to have children who also suffer from asthma. Almost all foods, clothes, perfumes, synthetic substances like plastics, natural substances like cotton, leather, pets and allergy to one's spouses can cause asthma. Allergens like pollens, flowers, molds and dusts always cause asthma in asthma sufferers.

Like other allergic conditions, asthma responds to Nambudripad's Allergy Elimination Treatments very well. In the beginning of treatment, it is always better to combine Western medical treatments with NAET to get better and faster results. After the patient is treated for the basic items, he can look at his symptoms and try to gradually reduce the drugs.

Asthma is not only a dangerous and distressing malady but seriously interferes with a person's ability to earn a living and lead a normal life. Therefore, patients who suffer from it should receive prompt allergic treatment. Since asthmatics can trigger an attack at any time, from any unexpected contact with an allergen, they should always carry inhalant sprays for quick relief in emergencies.

If not taken care of, asthma can turn into emphysema, in which, the elasticity of the inner lining and the air bags (alveoli) lose the elasticity. This makes it hard for the air to go in and out of the lungs freely. Oxygen exchange between lungs and outside air becomes difficult. The expanded air bags inside the lungs give the appearance of a barrel chest to the sufferer. These cases are usually far advanced. In the early stage patient can get good relief from NAET.

CHAPTER TWELVE

ALLERGY AND THE DIGESTIVE SYSTEM

The gastrointestinal tract is made up of the organs that have to do with eating and digesting food and include organs from the mouth to the rectum, which are part of the system. Therefore, allergic reactions which occur in or affect these organs, are grouped under the heading, "allergies of the digestive system."

Inheritance is a very important factor in this type of allergy. Like asthma, migraine, headache, hay fever, and skin allergy, they often occur repeatedly in families. Often the allergic history of a patient suffering from this type of allergy is found to be identified with that of a mother, father, brother, or sister. Even allergies to individual items such as milk, eggs, fish or onion may occur in two to four successive generations.

Gastrointestinal allergy is usually caused by foods, even though not all food allergies affect the gastrointestinal tract. Eggs, for example, may cause hives, skin rashes, asthma, or headaches, rather than an allergy of the digestive system. Allergy of the gastrointestinal tract may cause cold sores, fever blisters on the lips, canker sores, swelling and burning of the mouth and tongue, bloating, belching, sour stomach, nausea, vomiting, diarrhea, colitis, constipation, indigestion, infant colic, gall bladder symptoms, ulcer like symptoms of the stomach and duodenum, symptoms mimicking appendicitis, or any other abdominal conditions. Because the symptoms of certain allergic manifestations are so similar to cholecystitis (inflammation of the gall bladder), appendicitis, ulcers, and other abdominal diseases, many patients have undergone needless operations, causing much needless suffering and expense. And, unfortunately, they often do not reveal the true cause of the "symptoms." Consequently, they usually recur soon after the patient has recovered from the operation, and sometimes even sooner, leaving him in worse condition than before.

Such a case was seen by another allergist, and might be useful in giving the reader insight into the process. A woman who suffered from an allergic condition was diagnosed as having chronic cholecystitis, chronic gall stones and chronic appendicitis. She was also suffering from asthma and hay fever. The surgeon did not recognize the relationship between these conditions and her abdominal pain. She was operated on based on her abdominal symptoms and, although no gall stones were found and her gall bladder was normal, it was removed. Her attacks of excruciating pain in the gall bladder region, accompanied by intense headaches and vomiting of huge quantities of mucus mixed with bile, continued to occur at intervals of about one month.

After suffering from these symptoms for nearly two more years, she again underwent surgery, only to find that no gallstones were present this time either. The symptoms continued to grow more severe, with shorter intervals of freedom from pain. For eleven years this patient was completely disabled and confined to her bed most of the time, with almost constant and extremely severe pain. During this period, she underwent five major operations because of intense pain in the gall bladder region. After eleven years, she was almost never free from pain and required hypodermic injections of morphine two or three times weekly.

During these years, this patient had been under the care of more than a dozen different physicians at various times, all of whom treated her for the gall bladder pain either by surgery or with injections of morphine. None of them, with the exception of the last surgeon who referred her to an allergist, considered her symptoms of hay fever and asthma in relation to her other symptoms. None of them saw any connections between the gall bladder pain and these allergic symptoms. The dose of morphine required to relieve her pain had been gradually increased until she was receiving such large quantities that she was considered by some of her physicians to be a narcotics addict. None of them ever attempted to relieve her symptoms by adrenalin, until she came under the care of an allergist, who used this drug and so was able to relieve her pain without narcotics.

Because of this patient's condition, an insurance company paid for her complete disability over this period of eleven years. At the end of that time, she again requested a surgeon to operate because of the constant pain. However, he recognized her condition as an allergy, and referred her to an allergist, where she was tested for various allergens and was found to be sensitive to several foods, most important of which were fish, cheese, oranges, spinach, and wheat. She was also found to be allergic to various inhalants, like pollens and dust. She was treated by desensitization treatments for the known allergens. Her symptoms began to lessen gradually, and she was enjoying periods of several days which were entirely free from pain.

Within a short time after this, she made a final settlement with the insurance company, whose agent and the medical examiner could scarcely recognize the patient as the same woman to whom they had been paying full disability all these years. Eventually she was able to do her own housework again, and no longer received morphine injections. Although she was well past forty, she secured a job in the aircraft factory. There she was able to work her regular shift of eight hours or longer, although several doctors had given it as their opinion that she was totally and permanently disabled and would never again be able to do her own housework.

When it was realized that the same type of mucous cells form the lining of the gall bladder and its ducts opening into the intestines as occur in the nose, throat, and bronchial tubes, it can be readily understood why a severe allergic reaction of the gall bladder can cause the production of the same type of mucus as occurs in the nose, throat, and bronchial tubes. Spasms of the gall bladder and its ducts, as well as other parts of the gastrointestinal tract occur in the same manner as the spasms of the bronchial tubes which occur in asthma.

Unfortunately, in gastrointestinal allergy as in migraine headaches and some other allergic conditions, neither skin tests nor intradermal tests are infallible in determining the patient's sensitivities. Therefore, the causes of many cases of the food allergy cannot be determined nor treated by Western medical allergists. In such cases muscle response testing is the only means of diagnosing the allergies. Elimination diets or any other testing methods are not helpful.

In another similar case, a woman in her thirties was seen in our office. She complained of severe pain under the gall bladder region and numbness of the whole left side. Sometimes pain and discomfort under the diaphragm was her other complaint. She also experienced severe premenstrual bloating of the abdomen, indigestion, a feeing of a lump in the throat and frequent hypoglycemic attacks. She also had repeated Bell's palsy on the right side of the face. She could not close her eyes or talk properly.

This patient was operated on, and the gall bladder was removed two years ago. Luckily, she had only one surgery, unlike the previous case. She was found to be allergic to corn, wheat, eggs, meats, sugar, potassium, and milk. She was also allergic to cotton, polyester, and nylon. When she was treated by Nambudripad's Allergy Elimination Techniques, her pain started gradually diminishing. After six months of treatment, she is a new woman, without any pain or discomfort and hypoglycemic attacks. She still reacts to the substances as yet untreated but the reactions are less intense and of shorter duration. In addition, she has learned to test herself for the allergies through our monthly patient education seminars and is able to detect the allergens before using them.

Cornstarch seen in various foods, sauces, etc., is a very strong allergen and can manifest different symptoms in different people. As a rule, very few people are not allergic to corn or cornstarch.

A nine year old boy ate corn chips and got severe abdominal cramps and huge hives all over his body. Another patient, age 45, had constant breast abscesses, multiple joint pains, yeast infections, abdominal cramps and severe PMS, all from corn and corn starch allergy. Another nine year old girl had severe asthma all her life and was on breathing treatment every two hours, until she was cleared from an allergy to cornstarch. Many cases of migraine headaches got better after treatment for corn starch. A 28-year-old nurse complained of numbness on the left side of the body; a young man of 34 had blurred vision in spite of wearing glasses; and a 14 year old boy had frequent epileptic episodes. All of these cases recovered after treatment for cornstarch.

When infants are born, they are fed corn syrup and water from day one. It is no wonder then, that by the time they grow up they react to corn so intensely. We bring about our own sickness by eating the allergen beginning at a young age and by overloading the "toxin" in the body. Many arthritic symptoms are caused by corn and cornstarch allergy. Osteoarthritis, gouty arthritis, psoriatic arthritis, and so-called psychosomatic arthritis, respond well to the cornstarch treatment.

Canker sores, which are classified as an allergy of the intestinal tract, are primarily due to food allergy, drugs, and plastics in the case of dentures. Some people react to different salts and spices and these show up as canker sores. Practically any food may be responsible for canker sores, although eggs, chocolate, nuts, and milk, are very frequent offenders. They are quite often caused by one specific food item, as in the case of the man who developed blisters whenever he ate chocolate ice cream, which was one of his favorite pastimes. Another young man of

24 suffered from severe painful canker sores as an allergy to milk and milk products. Another girl of 15 suffered from severely painful canker sores together with hives, abdominal pain, swellings of the tongue and glands in the neck. In her case the culprits were eggs, and milk.

In many cases, canker sores are associated with other more severe allergic symptoms, as in the woman who also had severe recurrent headaches, gastrointestinal disturbances, acne, and almost constant canker sores for many years. Grapes and cantaloupes caused her problems, and she had made it a practice to drink a glass of grape juice every day since childhood.

Cracking of the lips and corners of the mouth also frequently occurs in cases of food allergies. Some cases of gingivitis (inflammation of the gums) and pyorrhea (inflammation of the gums with discharge of pus and loosening of the teeth) are a result of allergy to milk, iron, and vitamin C, although they may be caused by various substances. A 66-year-old patient ate some fresh avocado dip for dinner along with some Mexican food. An hour later, she had a severe toothache of the left upper first molar. She was allergic to the lemon juice in the avocado dip.

Food allergies may cause sore throat, or secretion of tenacious, adherent mucus. Patients who suffer from this particular allergic manifestation clear their throats frequently and sometimes almost constantly, hacking and drawing mucus down from the posterior nasal passages in an effort to relieve the feeling of congestion. At times, this congestion is so severe it gives the patient a feeling like he swallowed some large object which stuck in the throat and blocked the passages. Such patients often suffer from disturbed and restless sleep.

A 42-year-old female ate smoked rainbow trout at her friend's house. An hour later, while she was driving to her house, she began experiencing a mild sore throat. In two hours, she started to cough and she began having tenacious secretion in her throat that was hard to clear. She tried taking some antihistamines and decongestants at home. Even though she knew that the fish allergy caused this problem, she hesitated to go back to her friend's house to get a piece of rainbow trout, because they lived far away. But her postnasal drip kept increasing. In the night around 3 a.m. she woke up and started having difficulty breathing. This continued until 5 am. Then she would fall asleep for a while. Now 3-5 a.m. is related to the lung meridian. She coughed during the days and felt like she was suffering from a common cold. After nine days of struggling, she called her friends to make another piece of smoked rainbow trout. She was treated by NAET for smoked rainbow trout. Her throat cleared almost instantly. Within the next couple of hours she felt normal again.

Often sea or car sickness has been found to be caused by an underlying food allergy. People are very allergic to car exhaust, diesel, gasoline and their smell, etc., could be the cause of the car sickness. Allergy to salt could be one of the causes of sea sickness. Patients with a car exhaust allergy, could collect exhaust smokes from different cars and get treated by NAET. After successful treatment, such smell should not bother the person. There is an easy way to collect the sample. Get some wet paper towel and wipe inside the exhaust pipes of the cars and trucks. This will give access to the burned gasoline and diesel fuels. Also one should be treated for the fresh gasoline and other fuels too.

A male, age 36, suffered from asthma and Los Angeles syndromes. When ever he went away from Los Angeles, his lungs cleared, and he did not have much asthma. The moment he landed in Los Angeles, his chest tightened and breathing problems started. He was a lawyer by profession. He had to make lots of trips in and out of Los angeles. He was treated for automobile exhaust, gasoline, diesel, fire place smoke, and cigarette smoke. His asthma got better and he started liking Los Angeles.

The smell of natural gas burning could cause mental and emotional and physical problems. Cooking oil smell is another kind of fume allergic patients find difficult to manage.

A young girl was brought to Los angeles by her husband from a country like place in India. They lived in a small apartment. She started using natural gas for the first time in her life for cooking. They also used it to heat the house. In few days time she became very depressed, tired and slept almost the entire day. She had no energy or enthusiasm to do anything. She was unable to handle her daily housewife chores. Worried, her husband took her to different doctors. She was treated for psychological problems and placed on antidepressants which gave some relief. Then she started having severe nasal congestion, headaches and backaches. At this point, she was brought to our office. After elimination of few allergies by NAET, her problems were pinpointed to natural gas. When she was treated for natural gas by NAET, she became normal. She does not take antidepressants any more.

A 54-year-old female, could not distinguish the smell of fried oil all her life. Whenever she smelled any deep fried food, she ended up in an emergency room with asthma. She was treated in our office for heated oils. Now not only can she smell, she can also cook for the family and eat with them without getting any trace of upper respiratory problems.

Angioneurotic edema, a condition characterized by patches of circumscribed swelling of the skin, mucous membranes and viscera, is believed to be an expression of allergy. People with angioneurotic edema can get the attack any time. The throat can swell up making swallowing and breathing difficult or even fatal in certain cases.

A nine year old girl with complaints of swelling any where in the body is forces to stay home from school most of the time. She was found to be allergic to corn, spices, sugar, chocolate and fleece materials. After she was treated for these things her reactions became very minimal and rare.

An 18-year-old female had angioneurotic edema and her throat swelled whenever she went jogging or brisk walking. She was found to be very allergic to vitamin C, and citrus bioflavanoids. She was treated for vitamin C and bioflavanoids, and she did not get angioneurotic edema anymore. Soon after the treatment, she started jogging every day for a while. A year after the treatment, she joined the marathon and completed the 20 mile race with out any problem.

Anorexia (loss of appetite) is a common result of food allergy. This is particularly true in children, although it often affects adults. Nausea, vomiting, heartburn, and sour stomach are very frequent symptoms of allergy in the gastrointestinal tract. Most of the time, these are accompanied by hay fever, asthma, migraine headaches, etc.

A man who suffered from attacks of nausea, diarrhea and headaches after every meal was found to be allergic to the water he was drinking. He was also allergic to chicken, corn, wheat, and milk.

Another woman who had diarrhea every day all her life was allergic to the wheat that was her staple diet.

A female, age 48, had severe heart burn, sour stomach and frequent vomiting. She was allergic her own stomach acid secretion. She was treated for her own stomach juice and that was the end of her heart burn.

Severe intestinal flatulence could be due to poor absorption of the food in the intestinal tract. It could also be due to lack of intestinal enzymes, poor peristaltic movements, too much nitrogen producing food in the diet (dried beans etc.), or one may be allergic to basic or alkaline juice from the intestinal tract.

A male, age 44, had severe flatulence and bloating in the abdomen. No matter what type of food he ate, he was troubled with this problem. He ate only one food group at a time. He was told by a nutritionist not to mix different foods. He took different kinds of enzymes, before and after the food. Nothing worked. When he came to us he was a desperate man. He was treated with alkaline juice and relieved of his problems.

Some people could be allergic to acid and base in combination. These are the groups who are PH imbalanced. Their urine may be slightly alkaline and their blood may be slightly acidic. They need to be treated for acid and base together to balance their body.

Such was a case of 41-year-old female who was diagnosed as having candida, yeast, and chronic fatigue syndrome for a few years. She was unable to work due to her condition. She was on a candida free diet for years. She was found to be allergic to acid and base in combination; among other things like sugar, yeast, candida, grains, iron and coffee. When she was treated for the above items her condition changed toward normal. After four years of disability, she began working on a full time job and she felt okay.

Since the liver is the first organ that food proteins pass through after entering the blood, it is not surprising to find that allergic manifestations affecting the liver and gall bladder occur with comparative frequency. These manifestations are not necessarily identical, but may occur differently in different patients. For example, one patient suffered from enlargement and swelling of the liver due to an allergy to milk. Another patient suffered from enlargement and swelling of the liver due to an allergy to milk. Another patient suffered from intermittent low grade fever, which was also from an allergy to milk products. Another patient had his gall bladder removed because of severe abdominal pain which was later found to be due to apples and beef. Another man suffered from fainting spells, coated tongue, frequent urination, and mild angina pectoris (heart pains due to an insufficiency of blood supply to the heart muscles), all of which were relieved by the elimination of the offending foods. One patient who suffered from severe upper abdominal pains had her gall bladder removed to relieve the pain, subsequently she underwent two more abdominal operations only to find that the symptoms were caused by an allergy to egg and chicken.

Pylorospasm, which causes infant colic when it occurs in babies, is a spasm of the end of the stomach region called the pylorus. The contents of the stomach empty into the intestines through the pylorus which is surrounded by the folds of mucous membrane containing circular muscular fibers. When an allergy occurs that effects these membranes causing them to contract spasmodically, as do the bronchial tubes in asthma, the condition is known as pylorospasm, which is very painful. The pain in turn causes the child to vomit and cry almost continuously.

Such was the case of a boy, who experienced continuous pylorospasm and vomiting after each meal from the age of one week old. He also had severe colicky pains, continuous skin rashes, huge hives, ulceration of the gums, severe tongue coating, thrush, severe diaper rash, frequent colds and high fever, insomnia, and crankiness. He continued to have these until he was eight months old. His pediatrician suggested minor surgery to tighten the cardiac end, or beginning, of the stomach to prevent vomiting. Before he was scheduled for surgery he was tested by muscle response testing for allergies and found to be allergic to certain foods. He was treated by Nambudripad's Allergy Elimination Techniques soon after. At age 12 he is one of the healthiest children around. He can eat almost all the food he wants without getting sick. He does not get any skin problems, colds or flu. Incidentally, this boy is the author's only child, on whom she refined the Nambudripad's Allergy Elimination Techniques' success story.

In one case, the patient's abdominal distress was diagnosed as a gastric ulcer and even the X-ray seemed to prove the diagnosis. He was under the care of the best specialists available in a large city, who placed him on what was then considered a typical ulcer diet, consisting of large quantities of milk and cream with custards, cream soups, and similar foods. Among other things, he drank hot chocolate made with whole milk and cream, ate chocolate pudding, and was frequently served cream of tomato soup. The few meats and vegetables which he ate were ground to the consistency of baby food and were utterly tasteless. Under this regimen, his symptoms continued to grow worse until he was never entirely free from pain, carried a bottle of milk with him constantly, and was forced to take innumerable drugs to relieve pain and sedatives to relieve insomnia.

At last this patient was studied, from the allergic stand point, and was found allergic to most of the food items he was eating in the greatest amounts. They included milk, eggs, tomatoes, and chocolate, to name a few, and when they were eliminated, his ulcer symptoms were gone. However, although this occurred many years ago and he avoided milk ever since that time, this patient can still bring on an attack of abdominal pain and extremely bad breath by drinking a very small glass of milk or buttermilk. He could not even handle food made with a little quantity of milk at the time he came to our office. After being treated for food allergies by Nambudripad's Allergy Elimination

Techniques, he drinks three to four glasses of milk daily without any problems.

Allergy occurs with considerable frequency in the intestines where it usually causes symptoms of colic, cramping, constipation, diarrhea, soreness, and bleeding of the intestinal walls. Severe pain may occur as the result of an obstruction in the intestines by edema (swelling) of these organs. A tendency to bleed in various parts of the body is frequently present in allergic patients, as in the boy who had nosebleeds, bleeding from the rectum, or hemorrhaging of the conjunctiva (bloodshot eye) whenever he drank milk.

Constipation may also be caused by allergy of the gastrointestinal tract. The smooth muscle of the colon is a logical site for the allergic spasm and could very easily cause this condition. Since the intestines are lined with mucous membrane, it is also possible for large quantities of mucus to form here, just as it does in the nasal passages. It is even possible to have a type of contact allergy in the intestines because the food is in contact with these organs for a considerable length of time. In severe allergic constipation the muscle of the colon may contract to such a degree that very little food passes through this channel in a normal manner.

Since constipation is so frequently caused by food allergy, it is possible that many patients who load themselves with excessive amounts of bulk fruits, vegetables, bran flakes, and fibers in an effort to keep their bowels moving would have perfectly natural movements if their diets were studied from an allergic standpoint. For this reason, it is not advisable for allergic patients, or anyone else for that matter, to indiscriminately take laxatives. The very drug which is taken for this purpose may be aggravating this constipation. People who suffer from chronic constipation are often inclined to consider that there is little to be done other than taking large amounts of laxatives regularly. Actually, in many cases, the cause may be simple some food allergy which would clear up if the offending foods were eliminated.

A 34-year-old female developed severe itching and burning pain on the center of the tensor fascia lata muscle (a thick strip of long muscle on outer part of thigh). This muscle corresponds with the large intestine meridian. This lady was found to be allergic to all fibers that made her large intestine weak. She took psyllium seed and many other fibers very regularly. She was advised not to take a high fiber diet for few days. Her itching and burning diminished. Later when she tried to put the fiber into her diet, her itching and burning came back. At this point, she was treated for fibers and psyllium seed and her itching never returned. She now uses fibers and psyllium seed in her diet with out any discomfort.

Many people suffer from various mild forms of a GI allergy such as constipation, sour stomach, lump in the throat, nausea, canker sores, hyper-salivation of the mouth, bitterness in the mouth (especially early in the morning); fat around the abdomen, constipation, diarrhea, belching, bloating, dry mouth, extreme fatigue, sleepiness in the afternoons and so called hypoglycemic attacks. People with a mild GI tract allergy, do not take this into consideration and they may ignore the symptoms even though these symptoms have existed for years. However, a word of warning is necessary regarding the GI tract allergy. It can be serious and can lead to countless complications, some of which may even prove fatal.

Diarrhea, a condition which is the opposite from constipation, is also very frequently allergic in origin. It is often present in infancy and childhood and is frequently associated with colic, eczema, and vomiting. When the child grows up sometimes the allergy may become manifested strongly in other symptoms, and the diarrhea may get better. But there are cases in which diarrhea continues every day of a person's life until they die.

A 70-year-old female suffered from moderate to severe diarrhea for 50 years. She moved her bowels 10-15 times per day on the average. She was diagnosed as having pancreatitis. She also suffered from hypoglycemia for years. She was found to be allergic to all grains, vegetables, fruits, fats, sugars, and proteins. When she was treated for all these her 50-year-old diarrhea stopped and her hypoglycemia got better. At age 75, she enjoys her life better than she ever did.

When allergic constipation exists it may cause the intestines to retain the fecal matter (unabsorbed residues of intestinal excretions discharged from the bowels) until it purifies and so cause intermittent attacks of constipation and diarrhea. In some cases milk causes such severe diarrhea that even a few drops are sufficient to bring on an attack.

Very often both constipation and diarrhea occur in conjunction with other allergic symptoms as in the case of a 42-year-old man who had bilious attacks since childhood, migraine headaches on and off, abdominal pain and discomfort, mucous colitis, inter- mittent constipation and diarrhea, frequent canker sores, dry mouth, lethargy, insomnia, occasional hives, frequent urination, and bloody stools periodically. He also suffered from frequent colds and bronchitis and had a constant post nasal drip. He was treated by various medical doctors, including an internist, a gastroenterologist, a urologist, and a dermatologist for the skin rashes and hives. None of the treatments gave him any relief from his symptoms. Finally he was seen by an allergist who could not find any allergy to food items. The patient also had a pet cat. Due to his allergy to the cat, he was forced to give the cat away.

When he was finally seen in this office and tested by muscle response testing, he was found to be allergic to almost all the food items he was eating. He was allergic to chicken, carrots, peas, raisins, and a popular brand of tea. These were his major diet items. First he was asked to stay away from all the offending foods. In less than two weeks, he became symptom free. Later he was treated by Nambudripad's Allergy Elimination Techniques and he was freed of allergic reactions to the items and can eat almost anything now, rarely reacting to any food. He was also allergic cat hair and dander. He was treated for cat. Now he has another cat and can enjoy it without any problem.

Colitis is characterized by such symptoms as looseness of bowels, diarrhea, colic soreness, belching, vomiting, and varying symptoms of the stomach and intestines. Very often allergic in origin, certain types of colitis are caused by amoeba or bacteria. This type of colitis or dysentery is very common in the tropics and parasites are frequently brought into the country by returning travellers. In these cases, most of the time the parasites are allergens. However, the parasitical type of colitis is usually quite readily diagnosed by laboratory methods and when these tests are negative it is wise to consider the possibly of allergies as the etiology.

Another type of colitis, called nonspecific colitis, cannot be diagnosed by laboratory tests. This type usually occurs in nervous, excitable and unstable individuals and the nervous state is blamed for the colitis. Extremely nervous individuals are allergic to their own adrenalin. Usually extreme nervousness often accompanies, and very frequently aggravates, various allergic manifestations like colitis. These people are also very allergic to B complex vitamins.

A 38-year-old female always complained of severe diarrhea and severe perspiration of her palms before going for an official meeting. She was a bank manager and had several of these

211

meetings every week. She was found to be allergic to her own adrenalin. After she was treated for adrenalin by NAET, she never had that problem again.

It will be found that allergy to milk, wheat, gluten, and fruits will be the most frequent causes of allergic colitis, although allergy to vegetables, fish, meat, and other foods will undoubtedly be found to be responsible for the condition to a lesser degree.

Mucous colitis, the symptoms of which are very similar to those of ordinary colitis, differs from it in that large quantities of mucus are formed in the intestine and passed through the bowels of a person suffering from this condition. At one time this condition was known as "asthma of the bowels" and frequently occurs in people who have other allergic manifestations like asthma. The respiratory tract and the intestines are lined with the same kind of mucous membranes. Large quantities of mucus form in the respiratory tract when a person has bronchial asthma, and the same thing happens in the intestines when an allergy affects the bowels.

A 38-year-old man had suffered for several years with profuse watery diarrhea, associated with abdominal cramps and the passage of bloody mucus. He had mucous colitis. Some of his other symptoms were nausea, soreness in the upper abdomen, and a severe allergic skin condition. Careful laboratory studies and repeated examination, by various leading specialists, were made in an effort to determine the cause of his symptoms. But no relief had been obtained. When he came into our office, it was found that he had severe allergies to most common foods like beef, eggs, milk, breads, fish and fruits. He was treated for these various food allergies by Nambudripad's Allergy Elimination Techniques and in a couple of months he became symptom free and he could eat many of his favorite food items without any problems.

Another patient was repeatedly rushed to the hospital for operations because of suspected intestinal obstructions. Each time she reached the hospital, however, her symptoms improved before the operation was actually performed. At last it was discovered that her condition, which had been diagnosed as an intestinal obstruction, was angioneurotic edema (swelling) of the intestine caused by sensitivity to wheat. After the wheat allergy was taken care of she did not have the same problem. For some reason her brain was not releasing enough adrenalin when she ate the wheat, thus causing the swellings of the bowels. But when she was taken to the operating room fear caused more adrenalin secretion which took care of the problem.

Although all types of GI tract allergies are usually caused by food, some other substances such as inhalants, fabrics like nylons, flannels, wool, etc., may be also responsible for this condition. Another GI tract ailment, chronic ulcerative colitis, is also believed to be allergic in origin, food allergy being its main cause. Usually milk is the greatest offender, and most of these patients are sensitive to milk products. Other foods have also been found to be frequent offenders in causing ulcerative colitis. Probably a sore-like canker occurs at the site of a small lesion in the intestines and then becomes infected. When this occurs, a very large and excruciatingly painful ulcer is likely to develop.

In addition to various allergic manifestations of the digestive tract, many people suffer from mild allergies such as indigestion, dyspepsia, bloating, constipation, heartburn, flatulence, etc., which are not severe enough to send sufferers to seek medical help. Such people often take sodium bicarbonate, antacids, laxatives, etc., for the rest of their lives and treat themselves to relieve disturbing symptoms. Pain relievers taken for headaches, arthritis etc., may also cause GI tract irritation, so sometimes they do more harm than good.

In many cases of a mild gastrointestinal allergy, the symptoms do not become acute for many years. They might eventually get more severe with the patient often ending up having needless surgery. In most cases, if one learns to recognize the allergic symptoms early, the length of time of treatment can be greatly reduced. If treated before the symptoms get worse, the patient can avoid development of more severe manifestations.

CHAPTER THIRTEEN

ALLERGY AND THE GENITO-URINARY SYSTEM

As stated before, there is hardly any human disease or condition in which allergic factors are not involved. Further investigations into allergies and human ailments reveal new conditions caused by various allergic reactions. Any organ, group of organs, or portion of the body, may be involved and the allergic responses may show great variations. Causes of certain diseases previously unknown are now known to be entirely or partly allergic in origin. Bladder and kidney troubles, uterine dysfunctions, ovarian cysts, hormonal dysfunctions or malfunctions, premenstrual syndromes, infertility, cysts, tumors, infections of the reproductive organs, endometriosis, cancer, hypertrophy or hyperplasia of male or female reproductive organs, etc., may be the results of certain allergies and secondary effects of allergic reactions.

Many symptoms involving the genito-urinary tract are caused by food allergy. Food allergies should be checked first if someone comes in with an acute complaint of bladder or kidney infection. Such was the case of a 19-year-old female, married two months earlier, who came in with a severe pain of the lower back. The pain had started five days earlier, with fever, and severe chills for the past 24 hours. She had no complaints of frequent or painful urination, which ruled out the possibility of bladder infection. She complained of severe frontal headaches. Blood chemistry was normal. Urinalysis showed possible kidney infection. She was asked many questions regarding possible food allergies, but she could not remember ingesting any unusual food items prior to the onset of the backache. Finally, she was placed on aspirin every four hours, to relieve the fever, and ampicillin (antibiotic) to bring down the infection. She was asked to drink a lot of water and rest at home.

All went well, her fever and infection started to come down and she felt somewhat better. The third day she drank some herbal tea made of fenugreek. Within ten minutes she began to feel internal chills and had severe rigor in a few seconds, lasting almost forty minutes. At the end of the rigor, her temperature shot up to 105 degrees Fahrenheit, in spite of the aspirin and ampicillin. This time she immediately remembered drinking the herbal tea. Her husband tested her for allergy; the result was positive. They immediately came to the office and brought the offending sample. Tests in the office confirmed the positive result affecting the kidney meridian and kidney organ, and she was treated for the fenugreek. Her temperature came down to normal in 35 minutes after the treatment and didn't rise again. On further refreshing her memory, she remembered that she started using this herbal tea a day before the backache started. That confirmed our diagnosis that the herbal drink was the cause of the kidney infection which got better when the allergic reaction was removed.

A 49-year-old man complained of frequent urination for a couple of years. On certain days he had severe problems and he got up to urinate at least eight to ten times during the night, which made him very tired the next day. He had tried various treatments for this problem, including Western medical treatments with various antibiotics (none ever worked, he said), homeopathic medicines, herbal medicine, even straight acupuncture. None gave him relief. In our office, he was tested for food allergies and was found to be highly allergic to most foods. Placed on the program, he was treated for wheat, sugar, iron, vegetables, meats, milk, eggs, etc. His problem still continued and he was asked to keep a food diary. From this it was noticed that he was using a lot of artificial sweeteners. He was treated for saccharin, one of the ingredients in the artificial sweeteners, and he felt better for the first 18 hours. Then his symptoms started all over. He had lost the treatment (somehow the brain did not register the new knowledge). He was treated ten times consecutively, at the end of which he felt better, and the constant bladder irritation stopped. He is back to using artificial sweeteners with no bladder irritation.

A 46-year-old painter complained of frequent and painful urination, severe bladder pain, abdominal cramping, soreness, aching in the joints and extreme nervousness. Whenever he did not paint, he had no fever symptoms and when he went on vacation he did not have the complaint at all. In his case, the fumes from the paint caused his problem.

In some cases allergy of the urinary tract (to food or an inhalant), may also cause dermatitis and eczema of the genital area. The allergen is excreted in the urine and comes in contact with these organs where it causes skin allergies. Sometimes the anal region also gets skin allergies. In such cases, the irritating allergen is excreted in the stool. This was the case in a two year old boy who had weeping ulcers around the anal region. He was introduced to boiled egg as a daily breakfast item a month earlier. First, he had common cold-like symptoms for a week. When that stopped, he started complaining of pain while urinating and defecating. He had red rashes around the anus and it was very itchy. Parents were told by their family physician that it was the result of worm infestation. Since the family had visited one of the developing countries, the diagnosis was very plausible.

Lab work did not show any positive results for worms. He was treated for a month without any positive results. Finally, he was brought in to our office by the mother and evaluated. He was found to be highly allergic to eggs. Eggs were eliminated from his diet entirely. In 72 hours his wounds healed and itching stopped. Later he was treated for eggs by Nambudripad's Allergy Elimination Techniques. This boy was beginning to get some eczema at the wrist and ankle joints. After the treatment for eggs, even the eczema disappeared.

Another condition of the urinary tract which may be caused by allergies is hematuria, or blood in the urine. Such was the case of a 32-year-old man who had suffered for twelve years with severe headaches, nausea, vomiting, sour stomach, and belching. Later he also developed severe pain in his flanks, and for many months passed a considerable amount of blood in the urine. He also had a slightly enlarged prostate. All the tests, including a CAT scan, were negative except for blood in the urine. He was kept in the hospital for two months for tests and observation with no change in his condition. Finally he was sent home. A week later he developed swelling of both feet below the ankle, which made it difficult to wear shoes. His headaches got more intense, more frequent and he suffered from severe insomnia.

At this point, he came to our office for acupuncture to relieve his headaches. He was evaluated thoroughly and found to have allergies for wheat, cantaloupe, cucumber, and onions. Upon questioning him, it was revealed that he habitually ate one raw red onion with each meal. This practice started 12 years earlier, when he read in a health magazine that onion had blood cleansing properties and eating one onion a day could prevent heart disease. Ever since, he continued eating onions, which was the major cause of his 12-year-old health problem.

A 39-year-old woman had bladder trouble for 22 years, but skin tests did not reveal the sensitivities. She also suffered from migraine headaches. Since childhood she suffered from sinusitis and a runny nose. She suffered from feelings of burning in the bladder and pain in the lower abdomen, with frequent and painful urination. Sometimes she was unable to urinate, and she had to go to the emergency room or to the doctor's office to have urethral dilation. She always thought some foods affected her. Since she did not have any positive skin test for allergies and no one could do anything for her until she came to our office. She was tested and evaluated for food allergies and found that she was allergic to eggs, onions, potatoes, citrus fruits, wheat, cauliflower, cabbage, almonds, pears, cinnamon, alcoholic beverages, fabrics like cotton, polyester, and leather. When she was treated for these items by Nambudripad's Allergy Elimination Techniques, she got complete relief of her 22-year-old problems.

A young man who suffered from frequent and painful urination, as well as allergic rhinitis and hives, was allergic to eggs, beef, potatoes, tomatoes, and yeast. When he was treated by Nambudripad's Allergy Elimination Techniques, his six year old problem disappeared.

Enuresis, or bed wetting, which is such an affliction to the victim and to his family, is frequently caused by an allergy. A 13-year-old boy, who had severe enuresis and sinusitis, was allergic to wheat, rice, garbanzo beans, chicken, eggs, peppers, sugar, and gums. He was also found to be allergic to all synthetic fabrics. When he was treated for all these items by Nambudripad's Allergy Elimination Techniques he stopped bed wetting.

In a nine year old boy, oranges were found to be the culprit in causing enuresis. In another, a six year old, avocado, cauliflower, grapes, and cantaloupe caused enuresis. A 12-year-old girl who had this problem was found to be allergic to feathers, her comforter, oats, rice and yogurt.

Cysts in the ovaries is one of the common problems seen in fertile women. This was the case of a 32-year-old female who had frequent ovarian pains, which were discovered to be the result of ovarian tumors and cysts. Ever so often she had to take pain killers and antibiotics and most of the time she had to stay away from work. This woman was found to be allergic to soy and milk products. After she was treated for these products, she stopped having the painful attacks. Two years later, she continues to have no further incidence of painful cysts or tumors in the uterus or ovaries. Her severe PMS also disappeared.

A 35-year-old woman had an orange-sized tumor in her uterus. She had it for eight years but refused any surgery for fear that she would suffer the same fate as her sister, who died when she was operated on for a similar tumor in the uterus. This woman was found to be allergic to all green vegetables, fish, milk, beef, soy products, vegetable oils, caffeine, and chocolate. After she was treated for the above, she was placed on a special Chinese herbal formula to strengthen the uterus and remove the tumors. She woke up one morning and found herself lying in a pool of blood and in the middle of the blood was the orange-sized mass in the middle. She had passed it in her sleep.

Most yeast infections seen in the genital area are related to allergies. Most of the time, it may not be an yeast infection but some allergic reaction mimicking a yeast infection. If one could find the allergen, it would be easy to treat the yeast like symptom.

A 51-year-old female had this complaint for twelve years and was found to be allergic to cotton panties. Another 44-year-old woman was allergic to toilet paper. Another 31-year-old woman was allergic to the tampon and sanitary napkin she was wearing. After treatment, she stopped having the two year old nagging yeast problem. Another 41-year-old woman was found to be allergic to the decaffeinated coffee she drank every day. It caused a vaginal yeast problem. A 37-year-old man had a yeast infection and sores in the genital area for seven years, which was cleared after treatment for allergy to wheat and sugar.

Infertility is caused by allergies most of the time. A woman, 27 years old, was unable to get pregnant, even though she had been married at 19. She was found to be allergic to vitamin A, vitamin F, iron, B-complex, and chocolate. After she was treated for the allergies, she got pregnant within four months.

A 28 year old man had a low sperm count for four years. The couple had been trying to have a baby during those four years. He was found to be allergic to milk, fruits, vegetables, wheat, and vitamin A. He was treated for all these and he was advised to take "Shou Wu Pian" tablets (a Chinese herb to regain vitality and strength). Within three and a half months his wife was pregnant with his child.

A female age 32 suffered from severe endometrioses. She was married for twelve years and was unable to have a child. She tried various infertility treatments. Her husband was the only child of his parents. His parents were brainwashing him to divorce her and to marry someone else to get a baby. The husband did not want to do that because he loved her. This was why she came to our office. In our office, we found that she suffered from severe PMS due to endometrioses. She also suffered from sinusitis. She was allergic to many foods, grasses, pollens, cotton, polyester, and her husband's semen. After completion of the allergy treatments, she was sent to her gynecologist for possible removal of scar tissue from the abdomen. She was full of scar tissue due to endometrioses. After the surgery, she was placed on a special chinese herbal formula Tankuei and peony formula to regulate her hormonal functions. Within five months she got pregnant and they have a healthy beautiful girl.

Vaginal warts were found to be allergic in origin. In the case of a 42-year-old woman, cotton underwear was found to be the culprit. A 22 year woman had a history of vaginal warts for four years. She was allergic to soy products. In many people, elastic products can cause warts any where in the body which comes in contact with the products.

Say Good-bye to Illness

Another 62-year-old man had complained of severe and constant pain across the lower abdomen above the symphysis pubis. He had the problem for four months. He also had frequent urination. He was allergic to the expensive leather belt he received as a birthday gift four months earlier. When he was treated for the belt, his pain subsided.

Most prostatitis could be caused from an allergy to an individual's own semen. As men get older, as they accumulate more allergic semen due to less activity and the irritant semen causes irritation in the prostate gland. This can cause inflammation, and eventually even cancer.

An 84-year-old male was told that he had a bad prostrate and his urologist advised him to have surgery. He was treated for his semen, and when he went to his urologist for another check up in two weeks, his prostate was normal.

Many women suffer from premenstrual symptoms or syndromes (PMS). In some women, the problems start one week before the period and continues up to four or five days after. A series of health problems can be seen in PMS sufferers. Some of the commonly seen health problems due to premenstrual syndromes include: weight gain, craving sweets, craving salt, craving hot spices, bloating, tiredness, cramps in the lower abdomen, nausea, constipation, diarrhea, sore throat, sores in the mouth, dry mouth, dry lips, excessive thirst, excessive hunger, poor appetite, tearing from the eyes, temporo-mandibular joint pain, arthritis, frequent yawning, frequent sighing, night mares, dream disturbed sleep, body aches, itching, joint pains, headaches, stiff neck, back ache, pain along the spleen meridian, heart palpitation, fainting spells, ringing in the ears, hair loss, breast swelling, tenderness, secretion of milk from the breast, brittle nails, splitting of the corner of the nails, acne, painful boils any where on the face, mood swings, irritability, crying spells, anger, depression, sleeplessness, extreme sensitivity, thoughtless behavior, and even suicidal thoughts in some cases.

Some people get strange craving during this time. Sugar cravings relate to the spleen and stomach meridian blockage. These type of people can also have bloating, nausea, loose stools, soreness in tongue, sores in the mouth, painful boils or pimples on the face neck, heart burns and sour stomach, headache around the eyes and forehead, light, prolonged bleeding (8-10 days), dull cramps after the period starts, agitation over simple things, undue worry, and obsessive compulsive behaviors, etc., before or during periods.

Cravings to eat pungent food, craving onions, garlic, etc., is related to blockage in the lung and large intestine meridians. During or before periods, these types of people can suffer from mild to severe respiratory distress, asthma, colds, sinus problems, constipation before and diarrhea after periods, feeling sad and thinking about the past and weeping in silence, etc.

Salt cravings are due to blockage of the kidney meridians. One can experience thirst, crave salty foods, have water retention, frequent urination, headaches at the nape of the neck, fear fullness, etc., before or during the periods.

Cravings for sour things is due to liver and gall bladder meridian blockages. Pain and swelling in the breasts, pain in the inter costal muscles, severe abdominal cramps, heavy bleeding, severe mood swings, talking loudly, aggressive behavior, anger, and complaining are related to the liver meridian blockages.

Craving hot and spicy food goes with heart and small intestine meridian blockages. Heart palpitations, cardiac arrhythmias, insomnia, dry mouth, heavy sensations on the chest, night sweats, fatigue, over-excitement, insecurity, etc., can be caused from the blockages of these meridians before and during periods.

When the person craves these foods it signifies that there is a blockage in that meridian. If they eat the food craved in moderation, these food could help to open up the blocked meridians or strengthen those meridians. But if they eat excessively, then an imbalance of other elements takes place in the body due to depletion of other nutrients. This can increase the water retention, etc., causing more discomforts.

A 24-year-old female used to have itching all over the body that started four to five days before her period and lasted until the second day. She was found to be allergic to progesterone.

A 34-year-old female used to gain at least 8-10 pounds before her period. Usually after the period, she would lose all the water weight by the second or third day. She was found to be allergic to sugar and salt.

A 22-year-old female had severe abdominal cramps and severe indigestion when she started her period until she completed it. She was allergic to the sanitary napkins.

A 27-year-old female had nausea through out her period. She was allergic to the tampons she used. Another lady was allergic to perfume of the sanitary napkins, which made her very tired and caused depression.

A 32-year-old lady suffered from mood swings, crying spells, depression, insomnia, dry skin and breast tenderness before her periods. Once she started her period, she became normal.

A 26-year-old female had severe pangs of mood swings, depression, crying spells and arthritis around her monthly cycle.

Not only women, but also some men suffer from PMS and menopausal syndromes. Around certain times of the month some men become irritable, aggressive, agitated, moody or emotional and suffer from insomnia. This may be due to the hormonal imbalance or deficiency. Certain allergies also could cause these problems. One could easily isolate the problems through kinesiological testing and provide appropriate treatments.

Female patients who complain of premenstrual syndrome and associated problems like insomnia during their periods, tenderness of the lower extremities, tingling of both lower limbs, migraine headaches, etc., may have allergies to the sanitary napkins they are using. If they can change the brands or find a brand that suits their bodies (testing by muscle response testing) most people might avoid getting sick during this time. After avoiding all possible allergens, if they still have problems, the cause may lie elsewhere and they may need to see a specialist in the field.

CHAPTER FOURTEEN

ALLERGY AND THE CIRCULATORY SYSTEM

Diseases affecting the heart and circulatory system may be influenced by various allergies. Most chronic diseases do develop as a result of some chronic irritation. This chronic irritant could be an allergen. People who suffer from arteriosclerosis, or plaque in the blood vessels, seem to have allergies to milk products and calcium from very early childhood. When they ingest calcium products, the body does not digest, absorb, or assimilate them through proper channels. Instead, the particles get stuck along vessels and cause obstruction of the blood flow. Another allergic item seen among heart and circulatory cases is allergy to iron and iron products. Allergy to these two items, along with salt (sodium) and potassium, are seen among most heart patients. Cardiac arrhythmias, hypertension, hypotension (high and low blood pressure respectively), angina pectoris, allergic purpura, varicose veins and hemorrhoids are some of the diseases affected by allergies a large percentage of the time. Some hemorrhages caused by allergies may occur in various tissues of the body such as the skin, GI tract, eyes, nose, and urogenital tract. The people who are allergic usually bruise easily. People with varicose veins seem to be allergic to bioflavonoid (also known as vitamin P). When they get treated for vitamin P, and supplements are taken for a few months, varicose veins do improve significantly.

A young man, 38 years old, had severe varicose veins on both legs. He also suffered from bleeding hemorrhoids. He was found to be allergic to vitamin P. After he was treated for this, he was placed on vitamin P supplements. In six months not only did his hemorrhoids stop bleeding, but the varicose veins on his legs started disappearing. After a year he came in for a reevaluation. He had almost no varicose veins left on his legs.

A 60-year-old woman had varicose veins on both legs below the knees, appearing like a bundle of earthworms. Her feet were swollen all the time due to poor circulation. She lived in pain and nothing gave her any relief. She was found to be allergic to vitamin P. After treatment, she was supplemented with vitamin P, eight grams a day, and her pain and swelling decreased to a bare minimum by the end of a three-week period. After eight months of vitamin P therapy, she was evaluated and both of her legs were absolutely normal in size and free of varicose veins. Her legs were normal in color instead of their bluish earthworm-like appearance before the treatments.

Cardiac arrhythmia is produced by various allergies in any age group. A week old boy was found to be allergic to his mother's milk and had a heartbeat of 200 to 250 a minute. He was kept in the cardiac unit for the first two weeks of his life, due to the cardiac arrhythmia. Thinking something was wrong with his heart, his worried and anxious parents waited two weeks for the cardiac specialists to make a diagnosis to help with his problem. When the doctors could find no reason for the problem, physically or physiologically, his 22-year-old mother, who has some previous experience with allergies and the treatment using Nambudripad's Techniques brought the infant to our office. Sure enough, he was found to be allergic to breast milk. After treatment for breast milk, his heart started to beat normally.

A young girl of nine complained of heart palpitations one day around four p.m., after returning from school. Worried parents took her to her pediatrician and later to a heart specialist. She was found to be in good health. Even though she received a certificate of good health, she kept having fast heartbeats almost daily. She was seen in our office, evaluated and the history of her meal pattern for the week revealed she ate at least six to ten chocolate bars a week. She was found to be allergic to chocolate which was affecting her heart. She was advised to stay away from chocolate bars and her cardiac arrhythmia stopped. When she reintroduced chocolate into her food group the problem returned. Later she was treated for chocolate and she was able to eat it without producing any discomfort.

A 72-year-old female complained of cardiac arrhythmia and dizzy spells. She also had hypertension, severe arteriosclerosis, hearing loss, migraine headaches, abdominal cramps, swelling of both feet and had a mild to moderate amount of varicose veins. She was found to be highly allergic to cereals, milk products, chicken, turkey, eggs, sugars, vitamin A, fish, chocolate, vegetable oils, salt, caffeine, and various pollens and flowers. After she was treated for all the above items, her migraine headaches were completely relieved. Her blood pressure changed from 210/120 mm. hg. to 150/90 mm. hg., and it stabilized there without any support of medicines. She got complete relief from varicose veins and swelling of her feet. She also got relief from dizzy spells and cardiac arrhythmia. She did not show much improvement with the hearing loss.

A young man of 28 complained that he had low energy, no enthusiasm to do anything, and slept 12 hours a day. He had a low blood pressure of 80/60 mm. hg. and was found to be allergic to iron, salt, and sugar. When he was treated for these items, his energy level increased and he did not sleep more than eight hours a day.

A 24-year-old woman with an eight month old child began to experience frequent chest pain which radiated into her left arm all the way to the ring finger, at least two to three times a day. This began to get progressively worse. She was examined by a well known cardiologist who could not find anything wrong. She also began to get rapid heartbeats, off and on. One of her friends, who was previously treated for allergies by Nambudripad's Allergy Elimination Techniques, recognized her symptoms as allergic in origin and advised her to come and see us.

In our office she was evaluated thoroughly. It was revealed that she had just moved into a new house two months earlier where they grew a lot of tomatoes. They began to eat them, drink tomato juice (breakfast, lunch and dinner) and snack on them throughout the day. She was tested and found to be allergic to tomatoes. She took 11 treatments to clear her allergy, but afterwards her so called angina pectoris disappeared.

Most of the time, the causes of a heavy chest, chest pain, and rapid heartbeats are food allergies. Sometimes fabrics and jewelry can cause them. Such was a case of a 40-year-old woman, who had heart palpitations whenever she wore any synthetic materials or gold, platinum, and aquamarines. Being her birthstone, her husband gave her a set of jewelry with aquamarine set in platinum. Whenever she put the jewelry on she would experience heart palpitations and profuse perspiration. Once she was taken to the emergency room for the same complaints and they found nothing wrong with her. When she was finally treated for allergies to the stone and platinum, her heart started behaving normally and her perspiration became normal.

A 29-year-old movie producer moved into a new, expensive apartment. He began getting severe heart palpitations, severe fatigue, depression, extreme nervousness, nervous diarrhea, red and cracked tongue, rashes along the heart meridians. His problems started soon after he moved in but they got worse day by day. He suspected some allergy in the beginning and brought in all the environmental things from the apartment and the neighborhood like, carpet, wall paper, exhaust, grass, plants ceiling paint, etc. He was not found to be allergic to any of these things. Not knowing what is the actual problem, he had a complete physical including cardiac, and psychiatric evaluation. He even tried some counseling sessions. Nothing helped with his problems. He tried various treatments for a year. During this period, he became very sick. He was afraid to drive. He became almost disabled and sat in the house all the time. Finally the author decided to visit his house to see if she could find anything to help to solve the cause of his problems. She found out that he was allergic to all the built in wooden structures in the apartment. That was the only thing we had not tested him for. Little shavings of the wood were taken from the wood structure and he was treated. His one year old problem got solved.

Acetic acid is seen in a lot of hard plastics and many other products including nail polish, food products, etc., and is a common allergen that causes cardiac arrhythmia and heart problems which mimic heart disturbances. Another such item is the formic acid seen in most rubber goods. It also causes various ailments in the body such as extreme tiredness, chronic fatigue syndrome, aching feet, and tired eyes (soles of the shoes are usually rubber). Use of rubber, pencils, white-outs, etc., can also precipitate this syndrome.

Any allergies affecting the heart meridians and associated muscles are capable of causing disturbances in the conduction and function of the heart and circulatory system.

A 64-year-old man, who was recovering from a massive heart attack ten years ago, was told that his two major arteries were blocked 80-100 percent and he periodically had angina. He was found to be allergic to various foods, including organic and inorganic iron. He was found to be allergic to items made of iron, including the stainless steel bracelet he wore for religious reasons. It took eighteen treatments to clear the iron allergy. During the treatments, he experienced frequent chest pains, tiredness, leg cramps, insomnia, tingling sensations in various parts of his body, and frequent dizzy spells. When he was successfully treated for iron, his complaints diminished. Upon questioning him further, it was revealed that he was wearing his highly allergic iron piece on his body from early infancy for religious reasons. Wearing electromagnetic allergic field constantly for many years must have caused the blockages of the arteries and the heart attack. Since there are not many proven cases in this category, we need more evidence to support this theory.

Buerger's disease, which is a condition affecting the circulatory system, causes interference with the free circulation of blood, particularly in the hands or feet. In fact, the circulation of blood in the extremities may be completely cut off by means of a clot, which forms in the blood vessels on persons suffering from Buerger's disease, which is also known as thromboangiitis obliterans. It has been recognized that Buerger's disease occurs chiefly in heavy smokers and is caused by an allergy to tobacco, but it has also been seen with an allergy to aspirin.

A 49-year-old man had frequent headaches. On certain days he used 16-18 aspirin tablets a day to relieve his headaches. He also had poor circulation in his hands and feet and complained of pain in the distant limbs. He was a nonsmoker, but was found to be allergic to aspirin. Upon treatment for aspirin and clearing it, the circulation of the distant extremities was restored to normal.

The field of cardiovascular or heart and circulatory allergy is still quite new and hardly ever thought of by the treating physicians as compared to that of the more common allergic diseases. If more cardiologists were taught and trained to look for the connection between heart problems and allergies, more exciting discoveries could be made.

When coronary disease terminates life, the immediate cause of death is a coronary occlusion, or obstruction of the blood vessels that supply the heart, by a blood clot which stops circulation in the affected artery. If one could only investigate the causes of the clots and the causes of the heart muscle spasms before they occur, many fatal incidents could be prevented. The heart is composed of muscles and contains blood vessels just like any other parts of the body, and they can be affected by spasms brought on by allergic reactions. Therefore, it is perfectly logical to assume that angina pectoris, which is a spasm of the blood vessels supplying blood and oxygen to the heart, is sometimes caused by allergy.

A 44-year-old female who had hay fever, bronchitis, frequent pneumonia and hypoglycemia attacks since childhood was treated by Nambudripad's Techniques which almost rid her of her allergies. She was symptom-free and leading a normal life. One night, after eating barbecued chicken, she began to have severe chest pains which mimicked angina pectoris. She immediately tested the new barbecue sauce and found herself to be very allergic to it. She came into the office right away with the sauce and was treated by Nambudripad's Techniques. In a few minutes, her chest pain stopped. She had only one item affecting her heart so far, and that was the barbecue sauce. We could not isolate the ingredient in this case. Up to now, she has never come across another item affecting her heart.

A 66-year-old woman came in with severe chest pain after eating some food products given to her free by a senior citizens' free food service. White flour was found to be the culprit that had some insecticides sprayed on it. When she was treated for the insecticide her chest pain stopped.

A young boy who complained of frequent chest pain was found to be allergic to white potatoes. The parents of another boy observed that whenever he ate mashed potatoes he complained of chest pains. He did not react to french fries. The milk, butter, and potatoes combination brought on the chest pain. After he was treated for potatoes and milk products, his chest pain stopped. When his mother was tested for potatoes and milk, she was also found to be allergic to them, but she never manifested chest pains. However, she had frequent breast abscesses. Since she was treated for potatoes and mild her breast lumps have not returned. We can conclude from this that allergies are hereditary but are manifested differently in different people.

CHAPTER FIFTEEN

ALLERGY AND THE JOINTS

Arthritis is characterized by inflammation and pain in the joints. Joints of the body are found at the knees, wrists, elbows, fingers, toes, hips, and shoulders. The neck and back also have joints between the bones of the spine. Symptoms of chronic arthritis are pain, swelling, stiffness, and deformity of one or more joints. It may appear suddenly or come on gradually.

There are many forms of arthritis, the most common being osteoarthritis and rheumatoid arthritis. A degenerative joint disease is related to the wear and tear of aging and involves deterioration of the cartilage at the ends of the bones. The once smooth surface of the cartilage becomes rough, resulting in friction. The tendons, ligaments, and muscles holding the joints together become weaker, and the joint itself becomes deformed, painful, and stiff. There is usually some pain, but little or no swelling. Osteoarthritis usually develops around or after age forty. Approximately 15.8 million Americans suffer from osteoarthritis. It runs in families and more women, almost three times as many women as men, get affected.

Osteoarthritis has been found to be caused by allergies most of the time. Usually such cases are sensitive to food, especially wheat, nuts, spices, corn, gluttons, tomato, bell pepper, potato, salt, iodine containing foods like onions, turnips, sea weeds, string beans, chocolate, fish, citrus fruits, cheese, yam, peach, pear, and artichoke. Such cases are also allergic to dust, pollen, fabrics, and metals. Generally women do the cooking around the house and frequent exposure to different spices and food can make women more prone to osteoarthritis than men. Once again, arthritis is a hereditary disease, because of an inherited allergic tendency.

A 72-year-old woman came to our office complaining of generalized pain and discomfort. She was experiencing swelling and severe pains in multiple joints, especially in her hands and elbow joints, as well as in her hip and knee joints. She also had pain in her entire back. She was unable to bend over to pick up anything. She could not get up from a seated position without help. She had no allergies except that she had been asthmatic when she was a child. She was tested for allergies by skin tests which did not show any allergies. She was being treated by an arthrologist and took a great number of pain pills. She was tested for food allergies in our office and found to be allergic to almost all foods, but was not allergic to pollens or dust. She was also allergic to metals and fabrics. She was treated for the food items by NAET, one by one. At the end of two months, when she was treated for all the known allergens, she was almost 90 percent better.

A 23-year-old female student of nutrition was taught about the value of millet in the diet. She was excited to show this knowledge to her family. She went to a health food store, brought the millet, cooked, and ate the meal twice. The rest of the family ate it once that day. The next morning she could not get up from bed. Her joints were swollen and hurt. Her mother brought her to the office. Millet was affecting her joints. After she was treated by NAET for millet, her joint pain got better. Afterwards she was also cleared for wheat, corn, and barley. Arthritis was one of her complaints from childhood. When she cleared the grain, she cleared the arthritis.

Another young girl of 24, an assistant to a chiropractor, went to work one day and found she was unable to use her left arm. She had severe pain in her left palm and could not even hold a pen in it. The doctor thought she had stress fracture and offered to take X-rays. The X-rays were negative. In four hours time her pain decreased and when she went home her pain was gone completely. At home she ate a delicious corn bread left over from the previous night. In a few minutes the pain in her arm returned, this time more severely. She knew then that she was allergic to corn. Her friend brought her to our office to be treated for the corn allergy. She took three treatments. At the end of the third treatment she had no more pain in the hand.

Her history revealed that her grandfather died of a debilitating arthritis. Her parents both suffered from severe arthritis. Her 62-year-old father was almost crippled with arthritis. She was found to be allergic to most grains, spices, and citrus fruits. After treatment for all the known allergies, she was able to eat most of the food with out reproducing arthritic symptoms. Later she said that as long as she did not eat any allergic foods she did all right, but it she ever ate one allergic item that she was not treated for, she would immediately get joint pains and stiffness. She had no other health complaints.

Almost all the stiff necks seen in our office have contributing string bean allergies. Potatoes affect the vertebral joint in most cases. Spices affect the interphalangeal joints and wrist joints, and citrus fruits affect the knee joints in most cases. Corn, wheat, millet, barley, brown rice, oats and other grains affect all the joints of the entire body.

Rheumatoid and juvenile rheumatoid arthritis are types of inflammatory arthritis that attack the synovial membranes surrounding the lubricating fluid in the joints. The cartilage and tissues in and around the joints and often the bone surfaces are destroyed. The body replaces this damaged tissue with scar tissue, causing the space between the joints to become narrow, to develop folds, and to fuse together. The entire body is affected, instead of just one joint as in osteoarthritis. Rheumatoid arthritis creates stiffness, swelling, fatigue, anemia, weight loss, fever, and often crippling pain. It often occurs in people under forty years of age, including young children. Almost 2.1 million Americans are suffering from this disease.

Other forms of arthritis include gout, ankylosing spondylitis, and systemic lupus erythematosus. Gouty arthritis occurs more often in overweight people and those who eat rich foods. That's why it is also called "rich man's disease." This is also closely related to other foods, mainly iron, sulfites, beef, corn, and tomato have been the cause for gouty arthritis. In a young man of 26, tomato was the culprit behind his gout. A woman, 38 years old, was allergic to Mexican beans that caused gout. Yet another woman of 42 was allergic to her leather shoes which caused her to hurt like gout.

Osteoarthritis is mainly an allergy to calcium and milk. We had hundreds of people with osteoarthritis who got rid of their symptoms completely after they were treated for milk and calcium.

A young man of 18 was seen in our office for chronic, debilitating backache. His grandfather was a cripple at age 46 due to arthritis in his whole body. When the grandson began to show signs of early arthritis, he came in for allergy treatments. He was allergic to many foods and fabrics. His spine began to show osteophytic changes. When he was treated for milk and calcium allergies, his backache got better. He was treated for all the known allergies. Three years later when he was re X-rayed, his spine was cleared of osteoarthritis of the bone. Bone spurs can be removed by allergy treatments and supplementation with the proper vitamins.

Another 58-year-old woman complained of severe multiple joint pain and swelling of the joints. This moved from joint to joint at different times. She was allergic to salt and tap water and was treated for these items and felt better with her moving arthritis.

A few cases of rheumatic arthritis were found to be allergic in origin to foods and fabrics. After treatment for these items, the

237

arthritis diminished. A 43 year old female was diagnosed as a rheumatoid arthritic. She was taking many pain pills to get her through the day. When she came to our office, she still had swelling, pain, and stiffness of multiple joints. She was found to be allergic to some herbal tea she took for years to cleanse her body. After she stopped taking this particular herbal tea, her pain and discomfort got better.

Psoriatic arthritis is another kind of arthritis. Milk and milk products seem the worst agents for this kind of arthritis. A 72-year-old female had psoriasis all over her body and severe arthritis for 20 years. She was found to be suffering from psoriatic arthritis. She was eating cottage cheese every d
ay even though she never used milk in another form. After she got treated for milk and milk products by Nambudripad's Techniques her psoriasis disappeared and she got much better.

Another type of arthritis is called intermittent hydrarthrosis. This is a condition in which the symptoms are intermittent swelling and excess fluid in the joints. It may be recalled that typical manifestation of allergy are edema and production of fluids. This condition is caused mainly by foods, sometimes by fumes, pollens, etc.

Another kind of joint problem is called lupus erythematosus. In this condition, the joints affected are accompanied by general fatigue. The few cases treated in our office for his problem were found to be allergies to fabrics and materials rather than foods. A young woman of 28 was seen in our office for the possible treatment of lupus. She attended the lupus clinic regularly. She complained of severe joint pains and extreme tiredness most of the time. She said that lately the pain killers did not do any good. She had heard about acupuncture and herbal medicine and was in our office to find out if there was any chance to get any relief by having acupuncture and herbal medicine. Little did she know that we had something better to offer.

She was evaluated as usual and tested for all the allergies. She did not have any food allergies. She showed no allergies to pollens, grasses or trees. However, she was found to be allergic to all the fabrics and a few chemicals. She was wearing all cotton materials thinking that it was good for her. Surprisingly for her, it turned out that he was more allergic to cotton than to anything else. She said that about five years ago, at about the time she was diagnosed as having lupus, she found out that synthetic materials were harmful and natural fibers like cotton, were best for the human body. She discarded all synthetic materials in her household and replaced them with cotton, including sofa covers, and curtains. When she was treated for cotton, polyester, wood, nylon, acetic acid, formic acid, and tannic acid, her joint pains got better. Her energy level improved. A month later when she visited the lupus clinic, she was told she was under remission.

Another 46-year-old female suffered from joint pains, extreme tiredness, and asthma for the past 12 years. She was healthy and without any complaints before then. Her mother had suffered from asthma all her life and had died of it at the age of 44. The daughter had no sign of any allergy until she was 34 years old. She was tested and evaluated for allergies by four other allergy specialists and found to have no trace of allergies. She had to spend most of her time in and out of hospitals for joint pains and asthma. She was better within a day or so after checking into the hospital. Returning home, she started the wheezing in just a few hours. They moved to another house thinking that house was the problem.

In our office, she was evaluated and tested for allergies. She was found to be negative for foods, pollens, grasses, environmental items, hormones, fabrics, chemicals, etc. Her history revealed that she was married for 12 years. On questioning her further, she told us that a month after the wedding she got the first asthmatic attack. Searching her memory, she recollected her joint pains and tiredness started at least a week or two before her asthma. She was tested for her husband to whom she was highly allergic, but he was not allergic to her. She was treated for the allergy to him, which took seven days to clear. After she cleared allergy to her husband, her joint pains disappeared and her asthma also was better. She has not had to take medicines to control her asthma ever since.

Another interesting case is worth noting. A mother had three miscarriages and got pregnant again. This time she was extra careful and took all the precautions to prevent another miscarriage. She had severe morning sickness throughout the nine months. Finally, she gave birth to a healthy boy. Ever since she developed severe join pains and gained a lot of weight (40 pounds), even though she was a vegetarian and ate salads and low caloric food items most of the time. Finally when her child was seven years old, she was seen in our office and it was discovered that she had an allergy to the child which was causing the joint pains, tiredness, and obesity. The child was having some minor problems too. He was hyperactive, did not do well in school although he managed to get a B-grade average. He was very restless and had frequent nightmares, ground his teeth in his sleep, refused to make friends or take part in school activities or social functions.

The patient brought out another interesting fact. Whenever she slept with her husband and son in the same bed, she did not hurt in the morning as much as when she slept with her son alone. She became very sick with body aches, nausea, and stomach cramps. She was tested for her husband and no allergy to him was found nor him to her. This confirmed our diagnosis. When she was with her husband and son, the husband's strong energy neutralized the son's adverse energy, thus she was not affected. When she was alone with the son, his adverse energy affected her and in this case it showed up as joint pains. After she was treated for her son, she did not have any more arthritis pains.

This also made a tremendous change in the son's personality. He became more amiable, friendlier toward others, was able to study, and his grades got even better. He also stopped having nightmares and grinding his teeth, his relationships with friends got better.

These actual case studies show that arthritis and joint pains can be the result of any number of allergies. One should look into any possibilities like foods, environmental substances, animals, and other human beings. If one can trace the root cause, avoidance will give relief and treatment will give a complete cure and the freedom toady from the allergens without adverse reactions.

CHAPTER SIXTEEN

ALLERGY AND THE SKIN

Skin allergy is extremely important and includes many allergic conditions ranging from ordinary hives to severe atopic dermatitis or eczema. Skin allergies are visible to the patient and they usually receive more attention than any other allergic problem. When they clear up and the skin returns to a normal condition, the results are so dramatic and pleasing to the patient that allergy treatment seems almost a miracle.

Atopic dermatitis seems to be hereditary in nature. Contact dermatitis is caused most of the time by external contact with some allergen such as wool, cotton, polyester, other fabrics, cosmetics, etc. Atopic dermatitis is an inflammation of the skin which is often called eczema. It causes the skin to become patchy, with flat, reddish eruptions; occurring most frequently in the folds of the neck, back of the ears, on the wrists, the arms, the groins, back of the knees, on the bend of the elbows, and in the armpits. It occurs on the surface of flexor muscles (which serve to bend a limb or part of the body) and where irritation occurs through friction. It may occur on any part of the body, but almost invariably begins on one or more of the flexor surfaces.

When atopic dermatitis occurs in infants it is called infantile eczema, or "cradle cap" when it occurs on the scalp. As a rule, infantile eczema begins at about the age of two or three months and usually appears first in the form of a rash on the checks. In any infants it is limited to the face, scalp, and neck. Frequently, however, it spreads to the arms, trunk, and legs, and may become generalized over most of the body. The skin lesions are characterized by redness, blisters eruptions, oozing, crusting, thickening and hardening of the skin. It is often accompanied by intense itching so that the baby must have his hands tied or covered with mittens to keep him from scratching. Infantile eczema is usually caused by foods. In later life eczema can be caused by other substances like pollens, grass, fabrics, etc.

Contact dermatitis may be caused by baby oil, soaps, shampoo, clothing, diapers, laundry detergents, water, talcum powder, etc. One baby was six months old when she was brought to our office with infantile eczema. Her entire body was covered with eruptions and scabs. Between the scaling and blisters, made by scratching herself, this baby was a dreadful sight. She had her hands protected by cotton mittens. The mother had the baby clad in a cotton dress, cotton sheets, etc. Surrogate testing was done to determine her allergies. Since food testing by the computerized allergy tester, or any other method is not reliable for infants, surrogate testing comes in very handy. Her allergies were determined and the treatments started. She was found to be very allergic to vitamin C, milk, cotton, and polyester. Within a very short time after the causes were removed, her skin cleared up and she became a normal baby. The baby's paternal uncle had asthma and her maternal aunt had arthritis, hay fever, and migraines, all of which indicated a strong allergic inheritance.

Another infant, six days old, developed rashes, huge hives, and irritability soon after coming home from the hospital. The rashes got much worse and it was hard to put a diaper or any clothing on him. This infant was found to be allergic to mother's milk, cotton, and baby formulas. Since the mother had asthma, and she thought it was contributed by pollen, dust, etc., the house was kept very clean. When the baby was treated for fabrics, milk, and the baby formulas, the baby's skin cleared up very nicely.

A two year old was brought to the office with severe itching and hives. This child was allergic only to fish. The parents were very strict and never fed fish to the child. She drank only formulas, but the parents cooked fish at home almost every day. The smell of fish caused the dermatitis.

A girl, ten years old, had very itchy scaly skin on the back of both palms for seven years. Her parents had tried many different medicines and doctors to find some relief for the problem. She was found to be allergic to egg white and took seven treatments by Nambudripad's Allergy Elimination Techniques to clear it. At the end of the session her hands cleared. She was not fed eggs, but eggs are in a variety of food items like mayonnaise, salad dressing, cookies, even in some shampoos.

An infant who was three months old had a severe "cradle cap" itching and rashes on different areas of the body. This infant was found to be allergic to the wheat bread his mother ate every day, and he got the wheat allergy through the body. Most of the time infantile eczema disappears at three years of age. It may occur from time to time as different allergic manifestations.

A female patient was allergic to the peanut butter sandwich she made for her son every day. She developed deep furrows in the palm just by handling the peanut butter. After she was treated for peanuts by Nambudripad's Techniques her hand cleared within 24 hours. A 64-year-old woman had severe rashes and itching on her hand. For the past two days, her hands had many open wounds which started to weep. Upon questioning her, it was discovered that she bought a new water hose two days earlier and that was the cause of the dermatitis.

Alcohol is another item which has a strong tendency to cause dermatitis. A 50-year-old man suffered from contact dermatitis. He was treated for a few allergies with good results. He was very pleased with the appearance of his hands. He was suffering from allergic rhinitis and by next morning his dermatitis reappeared. After being treated for alcohol his problem disappeared and has not reappeared so far.

It is easy to trigger any kind of allergic reaction with any kind of substance. Therefore, it is best for the patient to learn to test himself before he buys clothes, groceries or any other items. Even if the patient has been treated for multitudes of things, he can still react to substances for which he has received no treatment. If he ingests these substances by mistake and does not get treated by Nambudripad's Technique or other means, the reaction can last on an average of three to twenty-one days. In some extreme cases, allergies from ingestion do not clear for years.

A nine year old girl ingested a special brand of peanut butter and an allergic reaction manifested as involuntary body jerks. At the end of three years, when the exact peanut butter was found and treated, her involuntary body jerks disappeared. This shows the allergic reaction can stay within the body for an unlimited time, even though in most cases it clears up in 21 days.

A 34-year-old woman had severe allergic rashes all over her face, neck, shoulders and scalp due to hair dye. After treatments, she could use the dye similar to the earlier one without any trouble. However if she used other brands she encountered problems.

A seven year old girl developed rashes every winter. She was allergic to the sweat suits she was wearing. A 37-year-old hairdresser had to work wearing cotton gloves for four years because of her severe, weeping skin rashes on both hands. She was allergic to the water at the place she had moved to four years earlier. Another housewife used fresh lemon to clean her silverware and developed dermatitis on both hands. She was allergic to the lemon. A 46-year-old writer had eczema on his right hand. He was found to be allergic to the stainless pen he was using.

Another man who had suffered the first attack of eczema at the age of five did not consult any allergist until he was 46. By that time his entire body was covered with atopic dermatitis, which had become chronic and had so thickened and distorted the skin that the scars are likely to be permanent. During this 40 year period, the eczema had gradually spread over the entire body and was complicated by hay fever and asthma. Unlike some cases of childhood dermatitis, this man experienced no lessening of the symptoms as he entered puberty. They remained present at all times and gradually increased in intensity.

When he finally consulted an allergist, he was tested and found to be sensitive to a number of foods pollens, and other inhalants, including animal epithelial, pollens, dust and the medicines he was using for internal and external application. After he tried traditional allergy treatments without positive results, he came to our office. He was treated for various food allergies, fabrics, and environmental substances. He showed marked improvements in his condition. However, the scars were so deep and of such long duration that his skin will probably never return to a normal state for years, even though he was absolutely asymptomatic. This is an example of neglected symptoms which are nearly impossible to correct. Had this patient consulted an allergist and received proper allergic treatment before the dermatitis became to severe, he would have cleared up the dermatitis entirely without leaving any scars.

Poison ivy and poison oak are both classic examples of allergens which can cause contact dermatitis. The response to these plants is a true allergy, since not everyone reacts to them, and many times prolonged contact does not bring allergic reactions. In other individuals one contact is sufficient to sensitize them.

A woman went on a vacation at a mountain cabin and there she contacted poison oak, which caused a severe reaction in her. She had severe itching, blisters and hives all over her body. She went to the nearest emergency room and got cortisone shots and antihistamines. She continued with this treatment for ten days.

She was still itching badly and could not obtain any relief with antihistamines. She was brought to our office, and in two treatments she was no longer itching or hurting. It took a few days for her lesions to heal. She made the mistake of breaking those blisters, which drained the lymph, and got infected. She had to take penicillin to prevent infection even after she cleared the allergy for poison oak. One has to be careful about the secondary infections which can be fatal at times. The primary cause may have been an allergy. If that is not taken care of the secondary infection takes over, and even if the primary cause is cleared, a secondary complication can linger on until it is also handled.

There are many people allergic to their jewelry, gold, nickel, and other metals. A 39-year-old woman developed asthma from using the jewelry cleaning lotion she used in her trade. A jeweler developed contact dermatitis to sulfuric acid which he used as a cleaning agent. Both his hands had deep wounds and he had to wear gloves all the time. Another patient, age 44, who worked as a hair dresser for twenty years, had a severe yeast problem. He was found to be allergic to human hair.

An unusual case of dermatitis, due to an allergy to fabric, occurred in a patient who developed dermatitis which only affected his arms. After a thorough investigation it was found that his dermatitis was caused by the mohair with which the arms of his favorite chair was upholstered.

Fur is often responsible for contact dermatitis and dyed furs are especially likely to cause this type of allergic reaction. One woman developed a dermatitis that first began on her face and neck, eventually spreading over her entire body surface. It was caused by the dye in the fur.

Stockings are sometimes finished with an alkaline substance that causes an allergic response in most allergy sensitive people.

When this is the cause of the dermatitis, washing will usually render the stockings harmless. But when it is caused by some synthetic such as those used in the manufacture of rayon and nylon stockings, good detective work is needed to find the cause. The same type of contact dermatitis may be caused by various articles of clothing made from cotton, wool, silk, or synthetic materials.

Sometimes the cause of contact dermatitis is so unusual as to seem almost unbelievable. Such is the case of a man who developed hives on his hands when his dog licked them. He was allergic to his dog's saliva. Dog hair caused no problems for him. An executive for a big firm, who spent many hours each day talking into a dictating machine, developed dermatitis around his mouth and on his right hand. He was found to be allergic to the plastic material of the mouthpiece, which he held in his right hand and pressed against his face.

A librarian, who constantly handled old books, developed dermatitis of her hands. It was found that she was sensitive to the glue which was made from fish products. Printers are very often sensitive to a fine lacquer type of spray which is used for drying inks so they will not smudge. Sometimes the sensitivity is to the spray as an inhalant and sometimes as a contactant. Regardless of the trade, profession, or occupation a person may follow, it is likely to involve contact with a wide variety of material such as dyes, chemicals, soaps, detergents, bleaches, plants, flowers, bulbs, woods, fabrics, varnished or natural wood, furniture, clothing, lacquers, rubber vulcanizers, foods, oils, greases, pieces, yeast, metals, drugs, metal polishes, celluloid, formalin, cosmetics, perfumes, and countless other substances.

Bakers are likely to become allergic to flour, sugar, palm or cottonseed oil. Barbers are very likely to contact quinine, resorcin, mercury, and sulphur in hair tonics. Dentists sometimes develop a severe dermatitis due to pain deadeners. Insect exterminators contact such chemicals as arsenic, formalin, sodium chloride and pyrethrum which is used in sprays and insecticides. People in the carpet business and furriers contact arsenic and paraphenyl enediamine, which are used in treating and dying the furs, as well as the treatment of animal dander. Gardeners contact various plants, arsenic, nicotine, insecticides, lime and fertilizers. Jewelers work with cyanide and sulfuric acids. Nurses contact bichloride, formalin, medicated alcohols, various antiseptics and drugs. Painters contact turpentine, varnish remover, varnish, lacquers, arsenic, linseed oil, aniline dyes and the lead which is in the paint. Printers are in contact with arsenic, artificial coloring, and hydrocarbons, in ink as well as paper, lead, and various compounds which are used to hasten the drying of the inks. Men who work in the tanning industry contact bichromate and hydrochloric acid as well as the skin of the animals. There are hundreds of others whose trades, occupations, or professions may bring them into contact with various allergens.

The acute type of urticaria (sudden skin rashes) can be caused from foods like strawberries and other berries, corn, cantaloupes, peaches, fish and shellfish. The chronic type, which sometimes persists over a period of several years, is more often caused by some basic food such as eggs, wheat, milk, oranges, chocolate, onion or other vegetables. Shellfish are responsible for a great many causes of hives. Such was the case of a young man who was very fond of fish, but got severe swelling of his face and throat immediately after eating it, then severe rashes all over the body within a few hours of eating. He was treated by Nambudripad's Techniques and now eats fish almost every day without any problems.

Another woman suffered from hives and severe migraines. The hives occurred mostly on the face while the headaches usually occurred after she ate. She was found to be allergic to almost all foods and fabrics. When she received treatment for most basic foods, she was cleared of her headaches as well as hives. When she was cleared of the food, she cleared the fabrics without any further treatments.

A girl, who was under treatment for hay fever and asthma, also had occasional attacks of angioneurotic edema. Among other foods, she was very allergic to turkey and after Thanksgiving dinner she got the worst attack of angioneurotic edema every year. She was treated for turkey. She did not get the usual attack after this year's Thanksgiving dinner.

Other skin diseases, which are known to have an allergic factor involved are dermographia, acne, pruritic, and psoriasis. A 72-year-old woman had severe psoriasis for the past 20 years. She was fond to be allergic to milk products and her lunch included cottage cheese every day. Her psoriasis cleared when she cleared the milk products. Another 20 year old psoriasis case was allergic to apples, and she ate one very day (to keep the doctor away?). After she was cleared for apples her psoriasis disappeared.

Acne usually clears with good nutrition after clearing the allergy for vitamin C, iron, zinc and vitamin A.

One has to be a good detective to find the allergen causing a particular problem. Identifying the allergens is usually the hardest part. Treatment is relatively easy. Various allergic manifestations of the skin are extremely important because of their influence on patients' lives. Anyone who is afflicted with a scarred, pitted, or crusted skin is handicapped both socially and economically. To this large portion of the population, allergy crimination brings new hope and the prospect of relief from chronic allergic skin conditions, which at one time were considered hopeless.

During migraine attacks, the symptoms may include any one or more of the following; blurred vision, blind spots, flashes of light, zigzag lights, blindness in half the field of vision in one or both eyes, intolerance to light, blindness, pain and a feeling of protrusion in the eyes, mental symptoms like confusion, light-headedness, forgetfulness, excitement, tendency to scream, cry or abuse, restlessness, irritability, slowness of though, difficulty in concentration, pallor, sweating, flushing, fever, numbness of the extremities, lips, tongue, nose, hands, or feet, diminished hearing, hallucinations of hearing, taste or smell. These symptoms are in addition to the severe headache which is present. Nausea and vomiting frequently accompany migraines and may last for a few hours or throughout the attack or may be absent entirely. Attacks may last from a few hours to one or two days or even a week. Following an attack, the patient may suffer from exhaustion, fatigue, loss of appetite and body aches, etc.

There are various controversial theories prevalent about the causes of headaches, especially migraines. From our experience in treating more than 500 cases of migraine headaches, over a three year period with 100 percent recovery by treating for allergies only, we conclude that the causes of migraines are solely allergens. Like anything else, it is up to the doctor and the patient to do the detective work to locate the offending items.

None of the existing modern techniques to test for allergies work to find the culprit in migraine headaches, because skin tests, scratch tests and blood tests for allergies are not able to diagnose food allergies. Elimination of foods from the diet is not efficient enough, especially when the patient is allergic to a majority of the foods he is ingesting. Muscle response testing is the only reliable method to find the allergen in the case of migraine, until researchers come up with another technique.

Many people have questions regarding the period of wellness between migraine attacks. The only hypothesis for this is that the brain responds to any kind of pain the body. When a patient gets a migraine headache, he experiences severe pain and the brain releases an antidote or a secretion that is a remedy from the allergen causing the existing migraine. The secretion is enough to neutralize the toxin and the brain secretes some extra amount and this lasts in the body for a longer period. During this time if the person eats or uses the same toxic product, the remaining secretion might neutralize it and cause no more attacks. Another possibility is the very foods that cause the trouble at other times are harmless to the patient in the presence of this neutralizing secretion. This is probably responsible for the cyclic or recurrent character of migraines. When this immunity or secretion diminishes, the body again becomes sensitive to the allergens and another attack occurs and the brain goes through the same functions again. This accounts for the periodicity of migraine headaches even when it is caused by such common food items as milk, wheat, eggs, chocolate, caffeine, etc., which are constantly present in most diets.

A 44-year-old female suffered from migraine headaches since childhood. She also suffered for years from seasonal hay fever, angioneurotic edema, severe premenstrual symptoms, etc. She went to a hospital emergency room at least once a week to get a pain shot and slept in a dark, noise-free room for two days until her headaches subsided. Nobody ever suspected or suggested the possibility of an allergy to this woman. When she came to our clinic, she was tested and evaluated for allergies and found to be allergic to almost all the foods she was eating. She was enrolled in our regular program. In two months time, her migraines were diminished. If she got one at all, it was from milk and lasted for a few minutes to a couple of hours. It got better just by working on the pressure points without taking any medicines at all. After seven additional months of treatments she was discharged -- nearly free from migraines. In the last five years, she returned only twice to our office with migraines which were of a low intensity.

The following is a very dramatic case of a migraine headache in which the causative factor was cornstarch and corn products. The patient ate corn and corn products at least two or three times a day until he got severe headaches constantly for nine months. He tried various treatments until he came to our clinic, and on our evaluation of history and symptoms, corn was found as the main irritant. He took 28 days of consecutive treatments by Nambudripad's Allergy Elimination Techniques just to desensitize him for corn. At the end of this period, not only did his nine-month old headache diminish, but he had also cleared many other food allergies he had prior to the treatments.

Another interesting case of migraine headache is worthy of mention here. Two days after marriage, a man developed a right-sided migraine headache. Two months later one of his friends brought him to our office. He was allergic to the bride. He was treated for her and after successfully clearing this allergy his two month old migraine disappeared. Luckily he was not allergic to many food items, but he was allergic to pollens and grasses. He had a history of hay fever since childhood, due to pollen and grasses, but had never had migraine headaches before his marriage.

Any chronic or acute unexplained headache, occurring periodically in an individual with a personal or family history of allergy, should be considered as allergic in origin unless proven otherwise.

Meniere's disease vertigo, dizzy spells, tinnitus (ringing in the ears) is a very common complaint mainly in older or immune deficient people. Some disturbances are due to swelling in the semicircular canals which are located on each side of the head, just within the internal ear area and are composed of three connecting canals through which the perilymph (fluid) circulates. These three canals are intercommunicating and lie in different positions.

On the inner mucous membrane lining of the canals are fine, very sensitive hairs or cilia, which are connected with the nerves and are constantly bathed in the circulating perilymph. This fluid moves from one part of the canal to another, depending upon the position of the body, just as a bubble moves in a carpenter's level. The semicircular canals control the balance mechanism of the body and it is through their proper functioning that an aviator can tell whether or not he is flying upside down.

Any disturbance in the passage of the fluid within the semicircular canals, any increase of fluid or swelling of the sensitive lining will upset the balance mechanism of the body and cause dizziness, staggering, or even complete loss of balance with falling or inability to stand erect depending upon the severity of the disturbance. In addition to prolonged and severe dizziness, inflammation and swelling of the semicircular canals, Meniere's syndrome causes such symptoms as nausea, vomiting, temporary deafness, and sometimes convulsions. Meniere's disease is often the result of allergies that cause swelling in the semicircular canals. Food allergies are the major irritants even though inhalants, sprays, fabrics, pollens, etc., can also cause it.

A 49-year-old woman suffered from Meniere's disease and was found to be allergic to her dear pet cat. Another 58-year-old female, suffering from the same disease, was found to be allergic to smoke from the cigarette her husband smoked. A 64-year-old woman was found to be allergic to the chocolate bars she ate twice a day. All these patients got rid of their disease after they were treated for the respective items.

But another patient, a 72-year-old female, was not so lucky as to find her problem with such ease. She was found to be allergic to various foods, fabrics, pollens, and inhalants. All of these items affected her balance. Finally, after she cleared for all the known allergies, she still kept having trouble with her balance. It was discovered that her hobby was tending her rose garden and she was found to be allergic to the perfume of the rose. After treatment for the perfume she finally got better.

Neuralgia is another disease of the nervous system often caused by allergy. It may occur in any part of the body, but is more likely to affect the head, neck, and shoulder. It occurs most frequently in patients who also suffer from other allergic manifestations such as eczema, allergic migraine, or GI tract allergy. The pain may be due to swelling of the nerves or nerve coverings of the nerves as the result of allergic spasm. Angioneurotic edema also may be responsible in some cases.

A middle aged woman suffered from severe neuralgia in the right shoulder, neck, right hip, and leg, which was associated with severe headaches, drowsiness, and sleepiness due to food allergy. Twenty two patients suffered from severe body aches and stiff necks whenever they ate string beans. Another lady, 34 years of age, suffered from neuralgia of the whole lift side of the body after she ate garbanzo beans in her salad.

Many people get neuralgia from allergies to certain bacteria and viruses. Such was the cases of seven females and three males of different ages that were affected by shingles which is caused by a virus. They all were allergic to the shingles virus. Their neuralgia got better as soon as they were treated and cleared of their respective viruses.

Epilepsy is one of the unexplainable diseases of the nervous system where allergy plays a great role. We had many epilepsy cases, all of which were allergic in origin. When they were treated for their allergies, they all stopped having epileptic attacks. Not all seizure disorders or epileptic attacks are from allergies, but if no other etiology can be found, allergy should be considered as a possible cause.

Say Good-bye to Illness

A 67-year-old man, who was subject to frequent epileptic seizures whenever he was standing in his backyard, was allergic to the new acacia palm tree he had planted in his backyard. A three year old female child was allergic to egg white which caused him to have seizure attacks whenever he ate an egg. A teenage boy got epileptic attacks once every two weeks, on Sunday nights. Every other Sunday he went to the beach with his father and ate a hot dog. He was allergic to the mustard on the hot dog. A teenager was found to be allergic to apples which caused the epileptic attacks. Another boy had epileptic attacks whenever he had chocolate.

Temporary paralysis is another disease affecting the nervous system. Most frequently the allergic attacks have been so great that temporary paralysis of a certain part of the body occurs. These symptoms usually disappear after a short time. However, if the causative factor is food allergy, it might last for long time until the same item is found and treated.

Pruritus, or itching, is a symptom which very often occurs as a result of allergy to foods or fabrics or chemicals. Pruritus is caused by an allergic response which occurs in the nerves which lie just below the surface of the skin.

A 69-year-old female came in one day complaining of generalized itching all over the body. Her history revealed that she had this itching all her life, but was worse in the last 22 years. She was told by many allergists that she was allergic to all the food items, environmental items and fabrics for which she was tested. She had various size rashes and boils all over her body. She weighed 67 pounds, was 5' 6" in height, and was very malnourished. On examination in our clinic, she was found to be allergic to everything including all foods, fabrics, and environmental substances. Her history also revealed that she had been very sick with whooping cough when she was an infant. Her parents and grandparents were quite healthy and died of old age. She could not remember any history of inherited allergies in their distant relatives.

She was tested and found to be very allergic to Bordetella pertussis bacteria and was treated by Nambudripad's Allergy Elimination Techniques for it. After successfully completing the treatment for pertussis, her itching diminished considerably and she was not reacting to most of he food items. She started eating normally and found she could assimilate the food without any pruritus. Her allergy probably began when her body's energy pathways were blocked with the incidence of whooping cough when in her infancy.

Insomnia is another symptom of the nervous system allergy. A 26-year-old girl suffered from severe insomnia, which kept her awake the whole night, while her husband slept like a log. She was used to having a glass of milk and a banana at night both of which she was allergic to and which caused the insomnia. Another patient, a 65-year-old woman had insomnia for 35 years. Upon questioning her further, it was discovered that she was allergic to vitamin C and she ate an apple, banana, or orange every night before she went to bed. The allergy kept her awake almost the entire night. Another woman ate fish every night for supper and had severe insomnia. When she stopped eating fish, she was able to sleep nights peacefully.

The field of nervous system allergy is still under study and we have not explored enough as compared to other branches of allergies like migraine headaches, GI tract allergy, etc. If we do enough research and detective work in this field, we will be able to trace a lot of mental and emotional disturbances as allergy based problems. Asthma, hay fever and hives were for many years considered to be nervous in origin. Now it is known that they are caused by allergens. In other words, an emotional upset may produce an allergic attack in an individual who is already allergic. But it is doubtful whether this ever occurs in the absence of an allergic predisposition. However, the nervous or psychic symptoms may be so pronounced, and the allergic symptom may appear so minor, that the relationship between the two is not recognized. This is especially true of a number of psychiatrists who blame all such symptoms on mental disturbances and rarely consider the possibility that allergy may also be involved.

Such a case was that of a 46-year-old female who was periodically very suicidal. Her friends were concerned about her behavior. They always kept her company. At a party one day, she got violently sick with an exploding type of headache and started talking suicide again. She refused to go to her counselor and her friends (some of whom had treatments for allergies by Nambudripad's Allergy Elimination Techniques) forced her to come to our office.

Her history revealed that her headaches began after meals. She was tested for various food items. One of her friends remembered to bring a small portion of the foods she had eaten at the party. She was found to be allergic to seven out of ten items she ate and one of them was affecting her brain. She was treated for this particular item and in fifteen minutes her head was clear and she experienced no headaches. She had been under psychiatric care for ten years. By then she was institutionalized for a while then she was released with the once-a-week follow-up instruction. She could neither hold a job nor live normally. After she was treated for wheat, sugar, milk, eggs, vitamin C, and meats she began to behave normally. Two months after her first visit to our office, she was able to work part-time which eventually changed to a full-time job. She went to see the counselor once a month and continued to live normally.

Another case was that of a schoolboy who had been expelled from three schools as incorrigible. He had severe sinusitis and hay fever, but this was not taken into consideration until he came to our office and discovered that he was allergic to various food items, materials and pollens. He was treated for all of these one by one and after clearing them his disposition changed completely. He got along well in school and in every way became a well behaved youngster.

Another young boy became mentally retarded at the age of two after he had been given various antibiotics to control his two-month-old fever. At the age of nine he could not talk or respond appropriately. He was treated for various food allergies and the antibiotics which were given in childhood. At the end of the treatment for antibiotics, this boy began to ask questions, engage in conversation and respond appropriately to questions. He was found to be highly deficient in B-complex. Supplements of megadoses of vitamin B complex helped in changing his personality toward normalcy.

Statistics show that eight million children in the United States suffer from some form of mental disorder. 1.4 million children are hospitalized for psychiatric care every year in this country. Could their disorders be due to food allergies? Symptoms of disobedience, surliness, irritability, and extreme nervousness are very often found in allergic children and even in adults.

Hyperactivity is another form of nervous allergy. Any allergen that affects the brain and nervous system can produce hyperactivity in children and adults. Foods, fabrics, materials, environmental substances, animals or humans can cause this type of allergy. Such was the case of an eight year old boy who was very intelligent but could not concentrate on anything. A child who was allergic to various foods was treated for almost all known food allergies. He felt better in regard to his hay fever and nasal allergies, etc., but his hyperactivity did not get better. Finally it was discovered that he was allergic to his mother, father, grandparents and his pet dog. He was treated for each one

259

of them. When he finished the treatments for his household members, his restlessness and hyperactivity got better. He became calmer and was able to get better grades in school. Another hyperactive two year old was found to be allergic to his mother. Treatment for his mother made him a calmer boy.

Children who are hyperactive and disobedient may be suffering from allergies in their surroundings and not foods. When left untreated they get worse. This may be one of the reasons children turn to drugs and alcohol in search of relief from the effects of energy blockages caused by allergies.

If husbands and wives were tested and treated for allergies to each other, if mothers and children, fathers and children were tested and treated for allergies, there would be more sound, lasting marriages, fewer divorces, more stable, mentally healthy children and more value added citizens in the future. There would be less crime, fewer people in mental asylums, fewer birth defects, less mental retardation, less disease in general and more peace and less fighting in the world.

Contaminated, polluted water can also affect the nervous system. Such was a case of a 48 year old psychologist who felt mental cloudiness, drowsiness, extreme tiredness and lack of interest in everything. She was finally placed on disability. Various medical doctors diagnosed her as having a yeast, candida infection, Epstein-Barr viruses, chronic fatigue syndrome, etc. Nobody suspected any allergy until after eight years of wandering at different medical offices and hospitals. She was found to be allergic to various food items and environmental substances. She felt better and her condition began to improve after she was placed on allergy treatments. She still kept having mental cloudiness and confusion. Finally she was treated for her source of tap water and filtered drinking water. Her mental cloudiness cleared and her emotional health returned to normal level after she was treated for the water samples.

A 46-year-old female became suicidal periodically. Her friends accompanied her wherever she went. She was also under psychiatric counseling for a year and a half and the patient herself decided to quit counseling sessions, saying she did not feel any better. When she was evaluated in our office, it was found that she was allergic to various food items, almost all affecting her brain, which made her suicidal. After successfully completing treatments for all her allergies, she became very normal.

We have had hundreds of cases of allergies affecting the nervous system. In almost all cases the patients changed from high-strung, jittery, emotionally unstable individuals into normal, calm, poised and assured persons. Each day our knowledge of allergy of the nervous system is being increased and it is hoped that the future will bring even more dramatic discoveries. However, our present knowledge has already brought great relief to patients suffering from this type of allergy.

Heat, cold, sunlight, and artificial lights are called physical agents. These agents have a great deal of influence on our lives and some sensitive individuals get abnormal reactions when they are exposed to them. This abnormal reaction toward physical agents also can be called "allergy." Most of the time this type of reaction occurs in patients with other allergic manifestations and may be divided into two groups. Contact reactions occur at the site of contact with the allergen, such as hives or rashes which develop on the portion of the body where the cold air or heat touches directly. Reflex like reactions may be more generalized or develop in the interior part of the body. An example of this type is the effect on the bronchial tubes.

A 72-year-old woman enjoyed eating ice cream. But whenever she ate ice cream she would get paroxysms of coughing or a choking sensation in the throat. When she melted the ice cream and drank it melted and warm, she did not have the cough or the choking sensation. Ice water also had the same affect on her. She felt uncomfortable in air-conditioned rooms with cold temperatures and got nasal congestion and a stuffy or runny nose when she walked in cold air. She was allergic to "cold." When she was tested for ice cubes, she was found to be allergic to them. She did not react to hot water or tap water. When she was treated for ice cubes, she found a tremendous change in her reaction toward cold and does not get throat irritation or coughs when she eats ice cream, nor does she react to an air-conditioned atmosphere.

A 55-year-old woman had just the opposite problem. She could not bear heat. She could not even drink lukewarm liquids which made her cough and her body turn red. When she walked in the sun she developed hives and red rashes all over the body. When she stood near a stove and cooked anything, she ended up having a headache. She was also allergic to various foods and environmental substances. After treatment for all the other tested allergies, she was treated for hot water which helped her to handle heat better.

A young man of 32 reacted to sunlight, but in a different way. He developed canker sores as well as skin cancers on his face, on which he was twice operated. He also had very many food allergies. When he was treated successfully for vitamin D and ultraviolet rays, his reaction to sunlight diminished. He was also allergic to the sun blocker he used on his body whenever he was exposed to the sun. After he was treated for the sun blocker, ironically his skin cancer did not return, and two existing spots disappeared.

It has been recognized for many years by various physicians that extremes of temperature, particularly of cold, may bring on attacks of asthma or hives. As long ago as 1860, a physician described attacks of asthma which were produced in a man by applying cold water to his instep. In 1866, another physician reported that cold water invariably produced intense hives on his skin. In 1872, a physician reported the case of a woman of 45 years of age on whom marked swelling of the hand could be produced by immersing it in cold water. The swelling subsided in fifteen minutes after reaching its peak. Cold air produced hives on her face and neck and the eating of ice cream immediately caused her intense pain in her throat and a feeling of suffocation.

Weather changes affect allergic patients greatly. Mainly arthritics and respiratory tract allergy patients are affected badly with high or low temperatures. When the temperature falls, the humidity increases and this affects asthmatics seriously, sometimes fatally. Change in altitude also can cause difficulties to allergic patients. Some people do well in high altitudes whereas some cannot tolerate it at all.

The cold may affect some people so severely as to cause fainting or loss of consciousness which may explain many deaths from drowning. Jumping into a cold-water lake can cause cramping and drowning, due to immobility and unconsciousness due to severity of pain. The fact that many such deaths of good swimmers has occurred soon after eating could be explained the following way. They probably ingested some food to which they were allergic, but which did not cause a noticeable reaction until a combination with the physical reaction caused a severe allergic attack. As in other types of allergic responses, physical allergy may be manifested in various ways. Some victims of physical allergy suffer from hives or angioneurotic edema of the hands when they wash in cold water. In others, the hives may appear on areas of the body which are exposed to the cold air. Some others may respond with swelling of the lips or spasms of the stomach following the eating of cold foods. Allergic rhinitis and asthma may be brought on by the inhalation of cold air. Some people turn blue in cold air and red under a warm sun.

Most of the time, low concentrations of certain nutrients in the body throw the body into imbalance and the body faces extreme discomfort when the weather changes. Lack of iron, vitamin B-12, and folic acid may cause poor quality blood, inability to circulate properly and thus block the ability to exchange oxygen and carbon dioxide properly. This causes more difficulties in extreme temperatures. Many patients who have extremely cold feet or cold hands suffer from poor circulation. After they take iron supplements, their circulation improves.

There are some extreme cases of patients with physical allergies. One patient complained of pains in the mouth, esophagus (the canal connecting the throat and stomach), and the stomach after drinking cold water. Cold air caused her lips and tongue to swell, made her eyes water, caused coughing and prolonged exposure caused asthma. She was treated for all the basic allergies to all the essential nutrients such as calcium, iron, vitamins C and A, trace minerals, salt, B complex vitamins, sugars, and fats. By the end of these treatments she no longer suffered from an allergy to cold air. When she cleared ice cubes, she was even able to drink cold water and eat ice cream.

Another patient, a girl, who was a victim of diabetes and kidney failure, could suck on ice cubes to quench her thirst (She was not allowed to drink water). She developed a chronic bronchitis and cough that did not respond to a series of strong antibiotics. After almost eight months of chronic cough, we tried to treat her for ice cubes. She took four consecutive treatments by Nambudripad's Allergy Elimination Techniques to clear the allergy to ice cubes. To our amazement, she cleared the cough and chronic bronchitis instantly upon passing the ice cube treatments.

Another patient suffered from hives, itching, and redness of the skin, headache, diarrhea, general weakness, and fainting spells whenever she walked in the hot sun, drank hot liquids or took a hot or warm shower. She was treated for hot water and has not reacted as much to heat since then. A woman suffered from severe asthma only in the summer and did all right in the winter. When she was treated for food allergies her asthma reaction to heat was reduced.

Very often physical allergies may exist in patients who are also allergic to other substances. While the physical allergy in itself is not sufficient to bring on an allergic attack, contact with the offending allergen plus the physical agent may precipitate an attack. An example of this type of allergy was seen in the woman who frequently suffered asthmatic attacks, which were produced by sudden exposure to cold wind. When the foods to which she was sensitive were discovered, and she was treated, exposure to cold wind also lost its effect. Sometimes people are allergic to both heat and cold, and this makes them miserable all the time. Such was the case of a man who developed hives and edema and sometimes dizzy spells after he played tennis. When he took cold showers he had similar complaints. He was also found to be allergic to various items including tennis balls, tennis rackets, shoes, soaps, shampoos, various foods, etc. After he was treated for all the known allergens, as well as for hot water and ice cubes, he no longer reacted to heat or cold.

Some persons are sensitive to the sun's heat only. In this case, they may be allergic to the sun's actinic rays only. These people also must be allergic to various items. In the presence of other allergies, an allergy to sun's rays brings on worse reactions. Such was the case of a man who worked on a farm and had severe dermatitis with redness, extreme swelling and itching of the face, lips, neck and hands. He could only work during the early part of the morning hours or late in the evenings. The rest of the time he spent indoors. He was also found to have various food allergies. After treatments for all the food items, his reactions to the sun were also reduced.

When physical allergy occurs in conjunction with pollen, foods or other substances, it is possible to treat the patients successfully by treating for the other nonphysical allergens. Most of the time, patients do not then continue to react to the physical agents. When people suffer from allergy to physical agents only, then they have to be treated for cold or heat. Such cases are very rarely seen. In these rare cases, when no other treatments work, it would be wise to avoid heat producing foods (according to Chinese nutrition theory) in heat-sensitive patients and cold-producing foods in cold-sensitive patients. The author has not seen, in her practice, cases that did not respond well to some kind of allergy treatments.

CHAPTER SEVENTEEN

BODY CHEMISTRY OR HUMAN ALLERGY?

We all know and talk about "body chemistry" and "incompatibility" in personal relationships. How did these concepts come into usage? Is there something like body chemistry and incompatibility, or could this be an allergy between human beings? Is this possible? Why not?

We know that we could be allergic to other substances. We could be allergic to other living things like plants, insects and pets. Everyone accepts this as a fact. Many people sneeze, faint and get hives in the presence of a cat or a dog. Animal epithelial and danders cause a great many allergic problems among allergic people. Saliva or other products cause allergic reactions in humans. If this is possible, humans could also be allergic to other humans, because each one of us has our own unique electromagnetic energy fields that can interact positively or negatively as with many substances. If these energy fields interact negatively, logic tells us it can lead to allergic reactions or discomfort in one or the other or both persons.

A 42-year-old female was having problems with her marriage for a couple of years. Joe was a devoted husband but could not make her happy. She nagged him and ordered him about all the time and insulted him in front of his friends. When she was alone, she loved him and regretted her behavior. They almost broke up twice during fifteen years of their married life. Now, for the third time, they were getting ready for a separation. During one of her office visits, the woman poured her heart out to the doctor. She said that she loved her husband so much that whenever she was away from him that she got physical pains just thinking of him. For some reason, whenever they were together, she irritated him and the days almost always ended in fights with the result that nights found them in separate beds. She also suffered from various allergies and manifestations like migraine headaches, gastrointestinal allergies and arthritis. She wanted to keep the marriage together but for some reason could not express her love to her husband. They had consulted a marriage counselor a few times but that did not help.

The concerned doctor asked her to try testing themselves at home by muscle response testing for possible allergy to each other. The next day these two were in the first group of patients. Their tests showed that they were allergic to each other, thus they both wanted to be treated for each other . They said that they spent fifteen precious years fighting and if there was a way to stop that pattern they wanted it to happen as soon as possible so as to enjoy the rest of their lives. A month later, after treatments for each other, there was a bouquet of red roses in the office and the note said: "Thank you doctor for helping us. We are going on our second honeymoon to the Caribbean; things can't be better between us." Six years later they are still in love.

A 28-year-old woman had three miscarriages and finally gave birth to a baby boy. She became very ill soon after childbirth with aches, pains, and severe arthritis. She was very thin and tall before childbirth, but soon after the childbirth she began to gain weight. In one month's time, she gained about forty pounds, even though she had not increased or changed her intake of food and had kept up with all her usual activities. This really puzzled her and her doctors as well. She joined an exercise program, which gave her some relief of her aches and pains, but not any weight loss. She tried all kinds of medicines and treatments, without positive result. The child refused to sleep in the crib, and the mother slept with him every night. When the baby got very sick, the woman's mother came and stayed with her to give her a helping hand with the baby. The child started sleeping with the grandmother. When the child stopped sleeping in the mother's bed, the mother started feeling better.

The grandmother stayed for a few more weeks until the baby's mother was well, then she left. The child started spending the nights with his mother again and in a few days she got sick again. Her arthritis and joint pains returned. Her fogginess of mind returned. She was lethargic and sick - even worse than before. Her worried husband took her to different doctors and tried all possible treatments. Nothing seemed to help her. Finally, someone guided her to our office. Her history was reviewed over and over. Her son was four years old by then and still slept in her bed. She was a very energetic, smart, slim girl without any health problems before the child was born. Now, all of a sudden, she was the sickest person in the world. Her morning fatigue and body aches gave us the clue. Again, when the grandmother stayed with her, and when the child spent most of his time with the grandmother, the mother recovered from her illness! When the grandmother left, and the child started to spend more time with his mother, she became sick again.

She was allergic to her son, as you undoubtedly have figured out. She treated for the allergy to the son and on completion of the treatment felt better, physically and mentally. She did not wake up hurting in the mornings. She also began losing weight soon after the treatment. She also shared with us more valuable information that she wanted to be included in this book, hoping it might help many other unsuspecting victims of allergy. She suffered from severe morning sickness and headaches, vomiting and nausea and tiredness throughout her pregnancy until the day of delivery. She was living on medication, one every four hours, throughout her pregnancy to keep her nausea under control. From this, we can form a hypothesis that pregnant women who have severe morning sickness and other pregnancy related sickness may be allergic to the fetus. The repulsion between the two energy fields may be the cause of miscarriages.

Many of the causes of infertility may be contributed to various allergies. If the couple is allergic to each other, or if the woman is allergic to the man's sperm, conception will not be possible. Infertile couples, who do not show any other physical or physiological abnormalities, should be checked for possible allergies. They may become fertile when the allergies to each other are cleared.

A 32-year-old female was trying to get pregnant for eight years. All the tests were normal with the couple. In our office they were tested for various things and found to be within normal limits. Finally, it was found that the wife was allergic to the husband's semen. After they were treated for the semen, within three months she was pregnant.

Another woman has been suffering from severe asthma for 15 years. She was on disability due to asthma when she came to our office. She was treated for various food allergies, environmental allergies, etc. Still her asthma bothered her every night. Finally she was found to be allergic to her husband. She made the connection between the 15 year old marriage and the 15-year-old asthmatic history. She was treated by Nambudripad's Allergy Elimination Techniques for her husband and her asthma left her.

Allergy to each other, allergy to husband and wife, allergy to mother and son, allergy to daughters, allergy to fathers, allergy to brothers or sisters, or to other members of the family, allergy between business partners, allergy between employer and employees, allergy between co-workers, allergy between teachers and students may sound unbelievable, but it is true as we have discovered. How many of us have seen once happy relationships end in fights and disharmony? How many of us have seen fighting between parents and simple arguments and friction between brothers and sisters, which when they grow up, end in severe fights and broken relationships? Many parents grow to hate their children and vice versa. How many of the most loving couples end up in divorce and hate each other for the rest of their lives?

Two siblings in their early fifties came to our office for allergy treatments. Even though they lived miles apart, they could not stand to be around each other for even a few minutes. They were like that all their lives, always clashing and fighting with each other whenever they met. Both had a lot of allergies to various substances and to each other. They were treated by Nambudripad's Allergy Elimination Techniques for all the known allergens, including each other. Now they are the best of friends, as siblings should be. They said that they are making up for lost time.

All of these external factors can turn into internal problems. If not taken care of right away they can cause severe illnesses. Each human body is different and each has its own electromagnetic energy field which is different from others. Therefore, it is quite possible to have a variety of results from attraction or repulsion between the energy fields whenever they come close together.

Astrologers talk about compatibility and we often wonder whether it is true. We have heard of people becoming ill after they are married or after living together in close proximity. We have seen people gain good fortune or even win a lottery with a jackpot on their honeymoon trip to Las Vegas. We also have seen some partnerships do well in business, in spite of all the odds against them, and some others go bankrupt even though both partners were hard-working and honest.

Similarly, we see a lot of our friends, who were in love, get married and in a few months hate each other and separate. Body chemistry and compatibility are not new to our vocabulary. But nobody can explain why these sorts of events happen. We call these behaviors of human beings by various phrases such as "lack of understanding," "cheating," "meanness," etc. If anyone noticed, and brought to the attention of others, that a healthy man took ill soon after getting married, a healthy bride became bedridden a few months after the wedding or after childbirth and died soon after, if anyone commented that his wife brought him bad luck -- these are nothing but the negative or positive effect of two charges between bodies. Just like other external or internal factors causing energy blockages, two different charges between human bodies can also affect the energy blockages and imbalances or diseases in one another. Or if the two charges are suitable to each other, they help to keep the energy meridians free of blockages in each other.

Some children suffer from various minor illnesses like hay fever, abdominal cramps, learning disability, lack of concentration, hyperactivity, etc. It is possible that these children are allergic to their parents or some other family members in the house. Such children could turn away from home looking for comfort elsewhere. Because they were allergic to their own parents, and they were suffocated in the house due to adverse energy, during the struggle to survive neither parents nor children understood what was happening to them. When the parents planned to have children, they had lot of pleasant dreams for the future. When the children are born, no one rejoices that occasion more than the parents. If the energy between parents and children is well matched, a lot of happiness comes to the house. Father could get a promotion soon after the child's birth. Mother could inherit a large amount of money or property from a distant uncle, because she was the only closest heir known to be alive when he suddenly died.

How many of you have heard or experienced wild but true stories like the one seen in "problem child?" We might say of course, that is just a story! But surely many of us have met lots of problem children. We have seen and witnessed many coincidental, unfortunate events in the past. We did not know what to think of it. The child in the movie "problem child" could have been born with an adverse magnetic force around him. If we corrected his adverse magnetic energy, he or his family and friends would not have suffered such misfortunes.

We have certainly seen events like this before. The father became unemployed as soon as the child was born. The father lost his hand or leg due to accident. While they were bringing the baby infant home, on the way from the hospital to the house they met with an accident and both parents died on the spot but the infant survived. The mother became disabled, due to post-partum complication. If the child's energy is very strong or adverse for the mother, the mother's life also could be in danger. If the parents' energy survived the child's adverse energy, after a while the father might find a job, the mother might come out of an acute phase of illness, their financial status might get better, but as the child grows up problems could be seen all over. Parents and the child might have small arguments in the beginning. Later on small arguments could get big.

Finally, the child would feel uncomfortable around the parents, he would begin to look for comforts elsewhere. If they do not find the right guidance and support with non-allergic people, they get into wrong company then into drugs and alcohol. Drugs and alcohol could give temporary false sense of well being. They might misunderstand and get into the addictive aspects. They could even leave the house and wander away looking for drugs and alcohol or looking for means to acquire them. Repulsion between the parents and children could be very small in the beginning. However, if there is an energy incompatibility, small energy differences could become larger and larger as time goes by, and it would increase in time and they could get into unnecessary, unpleasant arguments and fights. This may lead the children to seek shelters, join unhealthy groups and gangs, get into drugs and alcohols or get into self-destructive acts.

Say Good-bye to Illness

A seven year old boy was brought to the office seeking help for some of his allergies. He was found to be allergic to a few food items. He was also allergic to his mother and father and to the grandmother, who lived with his family. This child was also being treated for hyperactivity and behavioral problems. He always found some reason to argue and cry whenever he was with his parents. For example, "You don't love me, mommy, you hate me. I don't want to live in this house. I'd like to die. I wish I was never born, I wish I had another mother or father." His parents felt guilty and worried, not knowing what to do, because they loved him very much and did not know how to handle the problem. He was known as a wild child with a lot of bursting energy all throughout his infancy.

After he was treated for his mother, father, and grandmother, his personality changed for the better. He became quieter, felt very comfortable at home, began to express love toward everyone and even began to get good grades in school. He did not argue or fight with his parents unnecessarily after the treatment. The parents and this child were a few of the lucky ones, because they had the chance to discover his allergies in time before it got out of hand. His parents could breathe in relief that when he grows up, he will not get mixed up with drugs, alcohol or such unfavorable influences because he now feels secure and warm in his own home. His parents will probably never have to worry about him or his behavioral problems again.

A six year old male child was brought in with the complaints of hyperactivity. His mother also said that he was very destructive in the house, breaking and throwing things around and hurting his siblings. He fought with his older siblings all the time. He hurt his younger sibling and made her cry. The mother was afraid to leave him alone with his siblings even for few minutes.

She brought him into our office and he appeared very restless. He paced around in the room with out stopping for a moment. His mother kept telling him to calm down. He acted as if he never heard her, but he responded fairly well to the office staff. When he was with one of the staff, he was calm and responded to her questions. He was able to tell his name and he helped her to put a puzzle together. The moment his mother walked in to the room, his behavior changed dramatically. One of his neighbors, who had other children of his age, told us that he behaved very normal whenever he went to play with her children in her house. His mother thought that probably the cats and dogs in their house could be the culprit for this strange behavior. He was very allergic to sugar and trace minerals.

After he was treated for the food items, he still behaved the same. His older brother blamed the parents for giving him all the special attention. Once his desperate mother said sadly that she and her husband were seriously thinking of give him up for adoption, because he was destroying the family, and it was too much to handle him. He was found to be allergic to his mother, father and other siblings, as well as very many food items and environmental things. He was treated for all the family members. When he was treated for all the family members successfully, his behavior became normal. Two years later, he is a very happy, loving and smart boy and never gets into too much mischief. Now the parents are glad they did not proceed with their plans to give him up for adoption.

Another young woman began to have migraines a week after her wedding. She suffered severe migraines for twenty years and was then found to be allergic to her husband. She was treated and her migraines cleared up. Much unpleasantness might be averted if people would test themselves for possible allergies before they get into serious relationships. It is possible that in the future, when two people decide to get into a relationship or start a partnership, instead of going to an astrologer to reveal their compatibility they will visit a doctor who has knowledge of Nambudripad's Allergy Elimination Techniques to find out whether they are allergic to each other.

When people get treated for each other, they no longer suffer from problems they had. If everyone learns this testing method and checks one's allergies this can be a happier world, saving many marriages and relationships. There will be fewer runaway children and less drug addition and other bad habits. There could be more friendship and more love and caring among people, rather than enemies looking for fights.

CHAPTER EIGHTEEN

MISCELLANEOUS ALLERGIES

ACCIDENTS

Many accidents take place as a result of certain allergies. When the allergens affect the person's mind, or any part of the body, the body becomes weak and as a result accidents can happen.

A 42-year-old man went to the health food store to buy some almond oil to treat his dry skin, as advised by his nutritionist. He came out to his parked car with the bottle of oil in his hands, placed the bottle on top of the car, opened the door, got in and started the car to drive away. His wife, who was in the car, reminded him to pick up the bottle from the top of the car. He kept the bottle of oil at his right hand side, near the stick shift, and started driving.

This time, instead of turning right to get out of the shopping complex, he turned left which lead to a dead end. This was familiar territory to him, yet he made a mistake. His wife reminded him calmly about the mistake. He obeyed silently without any argument, unlike his normal self. Then he made a left turn into a one way lane going the wrong way and almost crashed into another car that was coming head on. His wife screamed in fear. Before he got too far, he made four more driving errors, which made his wife very suspicious. She knew her husband very well. If he had to drive blindfolded he wouldn't have made such mistakes. She knew there was something terribly wrong with him to behave like that. She immediately suspected the almond oil as a cause to his unconscious behavior. She threw the bottle to the back seat of the wagon as he was driving. When they reached home, he was tested for the allergy to the almond oil and found to be allergic. His liver and brain meridians were blocked with this allergy to almond oil. That was the reason for such confused and unconscious behavior! On questioning him further, he said he felt he was in a daze. He only distinctly remembered his wife's frequent screams at his driving on the way home. He did not even recall all his driving blunders. Almond oil had such an extreme effect on him.

How many accidents do we see on the road and how many of them are caused by these kinds of allergic reactions of the brain? The driver could be allergic to any material in the car, the seat, the wheel, the doors, the fabrics, the dust, fumes, pollutants, etc. They may influence the way he feels and, if the brain gets an allergic reaction, he might react unpredictably and cause an accident.

ADDICTIONS

Many addictions are caused by allergies, such as alcohol addiction. (We have explained this in an earlier chapter). Most alcoholics are allergic to sugar and vitamin B-complex. Craving alcohol is one way for the body to acquire sugar. When alcoholics are treated for sugar and vitamin B-complex, and supplemented with both for a few days, the craving for alcohol stops. Addictions such as sugar, alcohol, drugs, tobacco and overeating are caused by various deficiencies, which are in turn usually caused by allergies.

A 42-year-old lady, who was 60 pounds overweight, could not keep her hands off bread and rice. She was found to be allergic to B-complex and sugar. These caused blockages in the stomach and spleen meridians. After she was treated for B-complex, she no longer craved breads. She lost all her excess weight six months following treatment without dieting.

A 39-year-old patient had a case of severe hypoglycemia. She was treated by medical doctors, a nutritionist and some other holistic doctors with glandular therapy, etc. In our office, she was found to be highly allergic to sugar, carbohydrates, vitamin C, iron, protein and vitamin A. Her spleen, pancreas and heart were blocked. When she was treated for all these substances she stopped having hypoglycemic attacks. When she started eating normal foods, instead of the strict, hypoglycemic diet, she regained her energy. She was not sleepy in the afternoons anymore and could wake up in the morning without feeling tired. She joined an aerobic class, which was her favorite exercise program, and which she had not been able to do for the last five years. Eventually she became an aerobics teacher and does not have to fight hypoglycemia any more.

A 32-year-old patient was addicted to cigarette smoking. He smoked three to four packs a day. His wife was suffering from asthma and frequent bronchitis. Her doctor asked him to quit smoking for the wife's sake. He tried different methods to quit. He even went through a smoking withdrawal program twice; nothing worked. He was desperate. One of his friends was a smoker too and had quit smoking after treatment for his allergies through Nambudripad's Allergy Elimination Techniques and this patient came to us through referral. He was found to be allergic to B-complex, sugar and nicotine. His lungs, liver and large intestine were blocked due the above allergies. When he got treated for these items, he was able to stop smoking without any additional efforts. A couple of years later, when he brought his daughter to the office for treatment of allergies, he said that a week after the allergies to B-complex got cleared, his cravings for cigarettes diminished. He cut down his cigarette consumption, and in less than three weeks he quit completely and did not even miss it.

Addiction can be toward anything even toward a woman or a man. A 42-year-old divorced female fell in love with a married man. He spent a lot of time with her and told her that he was going to divorce his wife and marry her, but he never did it. Finally, this desperate woman told him to leave her and he did. In a few days she became very ill. She wanted to see him so much that she called him back. When he returned, he stayed with her for a few hours and she felt better. This pattern was repeated. Whenever he went away for a few days, she got very physically ill with joint pains, body aches, fever, etc. As soon as she saw him she felt better. Finally, she realized that she must be allergic to him and this allergy was turning into an addiction. She was right -- she was found to be allergic to him. Her liver, spleen and gall bladder were found to be blocked. She was able to break off with him without any repercussions after she was treated for him.

ALCOHOLISM

Alcoholism is mainly due to allergy to B-complex and sugar. Our body, especially the brain, needs a majority of the sugars we consume everyday for proper brain function. Sugar is necessary to produce energy in the body. When the body is allergic to sugar, the sugar is not absorbed through the digestive system via normal digestive process. Alcohol can be absorbed into the system through the blood stream. When some of the alcohol reaches the brain, it utilizes it for energy. The brain then issues commands to get more alcohol over and over.

People who are alcoholics, try to get more alcohol into the system on the brain's command. Momentarily alcoholics feel better soon after they drink. This is due to the action of the sugar increasing energy in the nervous system. When he drinks more, the depressive action of the "spirit" overpowers the body and the brain becomes sedated and weak. The brain starts functioning abnormally because of these factors. Most alcoholics behave soberly when they have some alcohol in their system because the brain will get some sugar to function. They will behave badly when they get too much alcohol in their system. When alcoholics suppress their desire to drink, they suffer from withdrawal syndrome. This can cause physical and emotional pain and physiological disturbances which are the brain's way of demanding alcohol.

Many people who go through Alcoholics Anonymous and similar groups will learn to quit drinking by practicing self control, group therapy, support systems, etc. But most of them end up having some physical pain like migraines, backaches, neck pains, shoulder pains, insomnia, etc. When they get treated for B-complex, sugar and alcohol their physical symptoms disappear. B-complex is essential for sugar digestion and absorption in the body, because most of the enzymes in the body are made in the presence of B-complex. If one has an allergy to B-complex, then sugar will not be absorbed properly. If one has an allergy to sugar, B-complex will not be absorbed. One has to be treated for B-complex and sugar before one can successfully get over a drinking problem.

Some people become alcoholics for different reasons: peer pressure, boredom, etc., or it is easily available. These people can drink any amount and rarely get drunk. These people fall into the non-allergic category. With a little will-power, they can quit drinking anytime without going through physical or emotional withdrawals or pains. Support and group therapy help, along with allergy elimination, to overcome addiction. Alcoholics are urged to join Alcoholics Anonymous to help break the long term habits and assure that they remain that way the rest of their lives.

A successful fiction writer, age 46, had to drink at least two or three beers before getting his flow in writing. Eventually, he started to become dependent on beer. It started to become a problem. On his wife's insistence, he joined an AA group. He quit drinking and also became very religious. Soon after he quit drinking, he started having severe low-back pain. He tried various treatments for his back for 15 years. He could not sit, stand or walk without pain. He lived on muscle relaxants and pain killers. He could not work effectively and changed jobs over and over; he would spend most of the time looking for jobs. When he came to our office, his history of 15 years of backache was unique. Upon questioning him, he said he quit drinking and immediately afterwards his backache started. This gave a clue to treat the items related to drinking. He was allergic to B-complex, sugar and alcohol itself. His kidneys and large intestine were the blocked meridians. When he got treated for these three items, he stopped having backaches. Five years later he still remains without any backache.

A 63-year-old woman came into the office suffering for two years with a severe strain in the left side of the neck, shoulder and upper arm. She was treated by a neurologist, an orthopedic surgeon and an internist. She was treated with physical therapy for four months. Nothing gave her any relief. She wanted to know what acupuncture could offer her. On a regular tongue examination, the doctor noted some signs of long standing addictions and liver damage. In the questionnaire she had not mentioned any addictions, only that she drank one cup of coffee, which was not unusual at all. This puzzled the doctor who asked frankly, "How much alcohol do you drink in a day?" She said,"I did not mention that I drank alcohol, did I?" The doctor said, "I know that. I read your statement. Now I want to know off the record, how much do you drink?" She turned pale as if she saw a ghost. She said, "doctor, how did you know that I was an alcoholic?" The doctor smiled, "Your tongue gave it away."

She said she was an alcoholic for the past 20 years. She even went to a "Stop drinking clinic" twice, but she could not do it. She worked for a telephone company. She was so dependent on alcohol, she had to stay home from work many times just for drinking. She hid the brandy (that is the only drink she used) under her bed. Her husband slept in another room and he never suspected that she was an alcoholic. She never drank in public. Her husband worked nights and she worked days, which made it convenient for her to drink. She never let on that she was an alcoholic. Even her family physician did not know. She faked migraines and got excuse letters from the doctor for work absences.

She was treated for sugar and brandy. She was not allergic to B-complex, which is why she could fool everyone about her drinking problem. Her large intestine was the blocked meridian. After she was treated for sugar and brandy, her nagging, constant pain in the neck and shoulder disappeared. Six years later, she still remains pain free. When asked about drinking, she said that she quit drinking soon after the treatment for brandy because she did not get the "buzz" in the head again. Brandy tasted like tap water to her after the treatments. She drank water whenever she wanted a drink since tap water and brandy gave her almost the same result. She thought she might as well drink tap water and save the money.

Fructose allergy can be a cause for sugar and alcohol addiction. Another alcoholic patient gave up drinking after she joined an AA group, but she developed very bad neck pains and bilateral elbow pains. She had taken up eating fruits and natural yogurt when she quit drinking. She was very allergic to fructose, which is seen in abundance in fruits. Fructose caused blockage in the spleen meridian. After treatment for fructose, her pains went away.

We have treated many cases of alcohol addiction, drug addiction, sugar addiction, chocolate addiction and tobacco addiction in the past five years. Almost all of these patients were found to be allergic to B-complex and sugar. As soon as these allergies were removed, it was easy to break the habits for most of them. Sometimes acupuncture is needed for three to four weeks, once a week, to bring down the cravings and withdrawal symptoms. During this time they are fed megadoses of B vitamins.

A 43-year-old truck diver was a known alcoholic. He wished to quit drinking, but whenever he tried to quit, he became very ill and could not do his job. After he was treated for sugar and B-complex, he was able to stop drinking alcohol. Whenever he craved alcohol, he ate some B-complex pills which helped him with his cravings. Eventually, he stopped having any more cravings for alcohol.

Some people do not get any unpleasant symptoms while they are drinking, but hangovers or migraines the morning after are quite common. These are the people who are usually allergic to alcohol itself. When they get treated for alcohol they do not get these latent symptoms.

A 36-year-old man woke up with a migraine headache every Saturday morning for ten years or so. Most of the time some over the counter pain killers helped him to get better. On certain days the headache got very severe. In those instances he had to go to the emergency room to get an injectable medication to help the headache. Other days nothing helped him. He had to sleep in a dark room for two days. He drank couple of beers with his friends after work on every Friday evening since he started his present job 10 years ago. Allergy to beer was the cause of his Saturday morning headaches and it caused stomach meridian blockage.

ANGINA

Angina pain can be caused by various allergens. Any allergen causing a blockage in the heart meridian could cause angina pains. Heaviness of the chest, pain in the chest, tightness in the chest, radiation of the pain into left arm and fingers, especially ring and little fingers, are some of the allergy induced angina symptoms. Plastic bags, and other plastic products, coffee, chemicals in the tap water, sulfites, fats, metals and spices are some of the common items causing angina like symptoms.

An 11-year-old boy bought two books from the book store. The books were in a cute plastic bag. By the time he got to the car, he began having chest pains radiating into the left arm and fingers. His father who was aware of the allergies and their manifestations. He tested him and found that the boy was allergic to the plastic bag and not the books, and the plastic caused blockage in his heart meridian. He took the books out of the bag and threw away the bag. In few minutes his pain and discomfort were gone. This boy was allergic to some chemical in that particular bag.

A 39-year-old woman had some dental work done in the morning. She began having chest tightness and pains by the afternoon. She was allergic to silver in the tooth filling. Silver was causing blockage in her heart and pericardium meridians. When she was treated for silver, her chest pains went away.

A 38-year-old woman had angina pain whenever she retired to bed. Certain nights she had to take 4-5 nitroglycerine pills a night. She was allergic to the materials in the mattress and pillow and they blocked heart meridian. When she was treated for those items she did not get the chest pains in the bed anymore.

ASTHMA

This subject has been covered extensively in another chapter. Asthma can be caused from various allergens that produce the blockage in the lung meridian or large intestine meridian. Food, drinks, environmental substances, animals, etc. can cause blockage in the lung or large intestine meridians and trigger asthma.

A 44-year-old woman had a history of asthma since childhood. She was found to be very allergic to bamboo. The bamboo caused energy blockage in her lung meridians. It was discovered that her house was decorated with bamboo and cane furniture. Upon enquiring further, it was revealed that her mother was also a fan of cane and bamboo. She had taken extra precaution to decorate each room with beautiful cane furniture. When she was treated for bamboo her asthma got better.

ARTHRITIS

PSORIASIS/ARTHRITIS

A 16-year-old girl had developed psoriasis on her scalp, elbow joints, knee joints and back and pain in all joints within a few weeks. This girl had taken a special liking to avocado lately. She was found to be highly allergic to avocado. Allergy to avocado caused blockage in the spleen and kidney meridians. When she was treated for this fruit, her psoriasis cleared up. Her joint pains also cleared up. Some of the shampoos and soaps also could cause similar reactions on the skin.

CHRONIC FATIGUE SYNDROME

This is a long term illness can affect the whole body. It is characterized by debilitating fatigue, and other persistent problems, such as low-grade fever, sore throat, insomnia or drowsiness, inability to concentrate, pain in the muscles and joints, enlarged or painful lymph nodes, general muscle weakness, headaches, forgetfulness, excessive irritability, confusion, difficulty in thinking, depression and lack of interest in life. Persons who suffer all of the above or some of the above symptoms fall into the CFS (chronic fatigue syndrome) group. This definition of CFS was developed by researchers and published in the March 1988 Annals of Internal Medicine. Previously, this illness was described as a chronic Epstein-Barr virus or syndrome (CEBV0) or chronic mononucleosis. Researchers decided that the name chronic fatigue syndrome would better reflect the major symptoms without suggesting a cause, because no one knows the cause of CFS.

In many cases, the cause of CFS is allergies to foods, chemical substances or environmental substances. Some people with CFS have an allergy to everything, including their own body secretions such as saliva, blood, urine and mucus etc. We see many patients with the above complaints who were going into CFS clinics for years with little result. When they are treated for allergies by Nambudripad's Allergy Elimination Techniques, they respond very well.

Such was the case of a young woman of 35 who was being treated for CFS and EBVS for three to four years. She was on disability for three years and was getting worse every day, in spite of all the treatments she received and good nutrition. When she was thoroughly evaluated in our office, she was found to be allergic to almost all the foods and fabrics. She was glad to know she was suffering from allergies rather than some incurable illness. In a couple of months from her initial visit, she started showing marked improvement. In her case, most of the allergens effected her spleen and heart meridians. She had four to six months of continuous treatment (three to four visits per week) to clear almost all allergies. At the end of that period she felt almost normal and began to work at a regular job.

A young woman of 28, who was being treated for CEBV for about seven years, was also found to be allergic to a great many substances, including foods, external substances, fabrics and water. In her case, she was severely allergic to regular tap water. She was also treated for her known allergies, which took almost a year of continuous treatment. She was on disability for seven years. Her heart, stomach, spleen, gall bladder and large intestine meridians were effected. After treatments in our office for almost a year, she was able to work full time as a teacher. Many mild to moderate cases of CFS were treated successfully with Nambudripad's Allergy Elimination Techniques.

Genetic predisposition may play a role in chronic fatigue syndrome just as we see in cases of allergies. Most CFS patients show inherited sensitivity to allergies. We are living in an environment of electromagnetic pollution. All types of energies are bombarding our bodies from all directions and cause continuous blockages. The result of this is a wide range of psychological and physiological disorders. Present day electromagnetic pollution may be causing weaknesses in the immune system. The pangs of immune deficiency diseases would not be felt so dramatically if one had a stronger immune system. Allergies will not affect the body so much. To strengthen the immune system, one has to strengthen the function of the thymus gland, the spleen, lymph flow and bone marrow. People who suffer from CFS and other immune deficiency syndrome ailments may be able to fight CFS eventually, if they make a point to follow balancing techniques twice a day.

Electric and computer radiation can cause energy blockages in the body. We see many people react to computer materials and radiation. We treat many people in our office for computer radiation. One of the many significant patients in our office was a 48-year-old male computer programmer, with extreme fatigue, frequent headaches, insomnia and irritable bowel syndrome since eight years of age. He worked as a computer programmer for eight years. He was allergic to computer radiation, which almost debilitated him from his normal life. Computer radiation effected his all 12 meridians. When he was treated with NAET for radiation and various environmental allergies, he was able to lead a normal life again.

DEPRESSION

Clinical depression is a much talked about subject now days. It is very hard to see someone normal anymore. Sometime or another everyone around us suffers from clinical depression. The increase in chemicals in our environment and pesticides in the food are some of the causes of the increasing problems. We are living in a chemical world. More and more chemicals are thrown into the world everyday. Everything we buy, may it be vegetable, fruits, grains, meat or cloths are treated with chemicals. It is mainly for our interest to kill the harmful bacteria, parasites or any other disease producing organisms.

This is also an era of science, a technological age. Science and technology have their place too. Many years ago, before the discovery of germs and germicides and antibiotics, we saw many lives were taken by infections and infectious diseases. Discovery of various medicines have helped us immensely to improve the quality of life. But the allergy to any medicine or chemical is possible just the way some people are allergic to natural foods. We need to recognize that and eliminate the allergies to the beneficial chemicals and drugs. Now we have an easy method to test allergies available through NAET testing. If allergies are found, they can be eliminated permanently too. There is no need to suffer the side effects any more. Running away from problems will not help us. How far can one run? Only until one meets the dead wall! Instead of running away from allergies, treat them and eliminate them. This will help one in the long run.

A 49-year-old school teacher suffered from severe clinical depression for a couple of years. She was seeing a psychologist regularly and taking antidepressants. Nothing seemed to help her. She was referred to our office and found to be allergic to grains,sugars, B vitamins, pesticides, make-up materials, detergents and soaps and they caused blockages in the stomach and liver meridians. After she was treated for the above items, she was asked to take large amounts (15 times the daily dosage) of B-complex vitamins. In few days, her depression was reduced immensely. She continued taking B vitamins for a few months. When her B-complex requirement was met, by taking large amounts for few months, she became normal again.

A 32-year-old registered nurse, who was our ex-patient, came to our office with complaints of depression which began one week earlier. She began crying desperately. She said she didn't see any need to live anymore. She felt worthless and unloved. Kinesiological testing revealed that the canned apples she was eating for a week caused her depression. The canned apples came from northern California from her mother's house. Her mother had canned them for her. In this case, she was allergic to the apples which affected her liver and caused blockage in the liver meridian. When she was treated for the apples, she had no more depression.

LATEX GLOVES

Latex gloves can be a very helpful item to most people. If the allergic person uses it, it can turn into a disaster. As we all know, many people are allergic to latex gloves. This is one of the common items in the hospital. Hardly any procedure is done in the hospitals without latex gloves. If the allergic person happened to use them it can be life threatening.

A 48-year-old woman went to a dentist to get some teeth cleaning done. The dental hygienist put on a pair of latex gloves and began cleaning her teeth. The patient all of a sudden began feeling very hot, her body became burning hot. The patient almost went into an anaphylactic shock. The doctor came and the emergency team was called. She was revived with the help of drugs. She had red rashes all over her body. She still had a mild fever when she left the office. She came to our office two days later. Red rashes were still on her and she was running a fever of 100 degrees Fahrenheit.

At that time, kinesiological testing showed she was allergic to the latex gloves the dental hygienist used. She was also allergic to the chalk powder in the gloves and they effected her large intestine, heart and gall bladder meridians. She was treated for the gloves and the powder. After she was treated for the gloves, she was also treated for local anesthetics, amalgam, cleaning agents, gauze and the cotton balls. She was advised to return to the dental office to finish up the dental work. This time she had no adverse reaction. She even had a root canal done.

Later, she confided that allergy elimination treatment for latex the gloves was the best thing happened to her in 15 years. Even though she was married, she was afraid to have intimate relationship with her husband for many years. She reacted to his semen and broke out in rashes and blisters all over the body when ever she had sex. She was allergic to the condom materials and couldn't use them. Later she was successfully treated for her husband's semen and she is a very happy woman now.

PREMENSTRUAL SYNDROME

Many fertile people, of both sexes, suffer from premenstrual syndrome. Even though males can also go through these cyclic changes, female PMS is the only one generally discussed. Hormonal imbalances from various allergies cause PMS. People with PMS are allergic to various substances. Some of the common symptoms are weight gain before periods, poor appetite or excessive appetite, headaches, tiredness, emotional swings, crying spells, general body aches, muscle aches, sleep disorders, frequent urination, constipation, dizzy spells or food cravings etc.

These individuals should be treated for food items like salt (allergy to salt causes blockage in the kidney and urinary bladder meridian and thus causes water retention), sugar (allergy to sugar causes blockage in the spleen and stomach meridian and thus causes bloating of the abdomen and weight gain), spices cause blockages in the heart, small intestine, lung and large intestine meridians. Blockage in the heart meridian causes the person to be overly sensitive, agitated, depressed, moody, easily provoked to cry, suffer insomnia and be highly irritable. Blockage in the small intestine may cause bloating, flatulence, poor sleep, night mares, etc. Blockage in the lung causes one to crave pungent and spicy food, have breathing problems, flu like symptoms before the period, high emotions, etc. Blockage in the large intestine causes constipation, diarrhea, abdominal cramps, heat boils or painful pimples on the face, neck, etc.

Some people crave sour foods. These groups of people may have blockage in the liver. They also may suffer from swollen and painful breasts, pain in the intercostal areas, excessive anger, migraine headaches (especially unilateral types). Many people suffer from allergy to sanitary napkins, tampons, chemical on the tampons, perfume on the napkins plastic wrapping, plastic lining,

292

cotton filling, etc. All these can produce premenstrual syndrome in an allergic individual.

Any of these items can affect any meridian, or part of the meridian, and could cause various unpleasant symptoms in a PMS person. Symptoms will depend upon which part of the body is affected. If PMS sufferers get cleared of all the basic allergens, and are provided with proper nutritional supplements, he or she will experience great relief from PMS within a short time.

EMOTIONAL BLOCKAGES CAUSING ALLERGY LIKE SYMPTOMS

A body should be balanced physically, nutritionally and emotionally. All of these three aspects are very important for normal health. If one is imbalanced, it can affect ones health tremendously. NAET doctors are taught to look at the body as a whole and administer the necessary treatments.

Emotional blockages can cause severe health problems. Emotional blockages could mimic allergies or various other common health problems. NAET doctors will be trained to isolate emotional blockages from simple allergies. They will also learn to eliminate emotional allergies and blockages permanently as the simple nutritional or environmental allergies. Let us look at some of the case histories of patients who had emotional blockages as primary causes for their health problems.

A 25-year-old woman was seen in our office for extreme fatigue, frequent fainting attacks, nausea, anorexia, sleeplessness, frequent vomiting when ever she ate sweets, and general body aches. She said that she frequently fainted as a child and vomited any time she ate sweets. She did not remember any trauma in childhood.

Say Good-bye to Illness

She showed emotional allergies to all the foods, especially to sugar and chocolate. Through neuro-emotional techniques (thanks to Doctor Scott Walker for teaching me this art) and kinesiological testing, it was discovered that she was molested by her neighbor when she was three years old. It was assumed that she was lured toward this child molester by chocolate candies and she was molested while she was eating candies. She may have responded to this unexpected attack with fear. She may have also fainted when he attacked her. She may have vomited with fear like many children do when they are frightened.

Her brain was confused at that moment because she was happy when she got the candy and when she ate it. But when she was attacked, she became fearful and unhappy. She still had the candy in her mouth. So probably her brain received a confusing message from the messenger nerves that eating sweet candy was the cause of her fear and unhappiness. The brain took note of this dangerous signal and with any future contact with anything sweet, the brain began giving signals about the possible danger to her health. This was the cause of her allergic reactions to all foods. She was treated for this emotional blockage with NET (Neuro-Emotional technique and NAET). After the treatment for this trauma, she quit reacting to food in general. Her fainting spells were gone. Three years after the treatment, while this book was being written, we contacted her and found out that she is a happy woman now.

A 46-year-old woman severely reacted to chlorox and bleach. An emotional allergy was discovered with this case too. When she was a new bride at 19, she scrubbed and cleaned the kitchen sink. Her father-in-law walked in and praised her saying what a good job she did, and he said that he wasn't aware that the sink could shine like that since he had never seen it like that before. Her mother-in-law stood next to her with a deep hurt in her eyes. She responded saying that she always kept the wash basin cleaner than that and he never bothered to notice it even once.

294

This made the daughter-in-law very unhappy. Ever since that time, she reacted to the smell or touch of any chemicals. When she was treated for the incident, she was able to use chemicals and detergents with out any adverse reactions.

A 59-year-old man had frequent headaches for a few years. His headaches were severe following any grain consumption. It was discovered, through kinesiological testing, that he had a financial loss when he was 41. He lost his restaurant business and was very sad about it. He may have been eating breads and grain products while he was grieving for the financial loss, and his confused brain assumed that eating the grain and grain products made him sad. Thus with any future contact with grains, his brain began giving warning signals as migraine headaches. After the treatment for the incident, he never got the usual headaches anymore.

A 28-year-old girl had nightmares and always woke up from sleep with fear. Then she couldn't go to sleep for many hours. Her dream was always around burning fire. She could not remember any childhood trauma or any event that her family talked about. She was living thousands of miles away from home now. Her parents were not living anymore. Through kinesiological testing, it was discovered that when she was six-months old, she was frightened by a scary fire. After she was treated for the emotional blockage, she quit having scary dreams and nightmares. She was puzzled by this childhood revelation that ruined many of her good years.

Finally she visited her old grandmother who told her that they had a threatening fire when she was about six months old and she was sick for a while after that. Everybody thought that she was sick from smoke inhalation, but she was in fact sick due to fear. We take it for granted that infants and small children do not understand anything. We do not explain to them properly if a disaster takes place. Their brain remains puzzled the rest of their lives. It would be a good idea if we had better communication with infants and children.

A 50-year-old woman was allergic to money. She was also allergic to many food and environmental items. She was treated for the allergy to money and that cleared all food allergies for her.

ENDOMETRIOSES

Endometriosis in women is found in increasing frequency, and no successful treatment has been developed so far in Western medicine. Many food allergies such as soy products, milk products, and poultry play a great role in this female problem.

A 28-year-old female patient had various treatments for endometriosis, including laparoscopy, a surgical procedure to clean the ectopic endometrial tissue. She suffered from severe premenstrual disorders, severe dysmenorrhea (pain during periods) and extreme tiredness. She was found to be allergic to a lot of food items, including milk, soy products and poultry. After she was treated for these products, her PMS and dysmenorrhea disappeared.

Another 25-year-old female was infertile due to endometriosis. she was found to be allergic to a lot of food items, fabrics and chemicals. Three months after she completed the treatments, she became pregnant. Even after the delivery, her endometriosis did not return.

EYE DISORDERS

Many times eye problems are a result of allergies. Certain food items that affect the liver meridian can cause eye problems. Conjunctivitis, red eyes, watering from the eyes, cataracts, and pressure in the eyes are all probably the result of some allergy or other.

A 51-year-old woman always had blurry vision. She had to change the power of her glasses often. She was found to be allergic to various food items and substances, including her contact lenses and eye glasses. When she was treated for all her known allergies, the power of her prescription came down and she does not suffer from blurry vision any more unless she eats some allergic food items.

A young boy of six had problems seeing and reading. He was taken to two different eye doctors and got exactly the same prescriptions for his glasses. He was found to be allergic to various food items, treated for all his known allergies, and in less than two months he started reading without glasses. He said he couldn't see anything with the glasses. He was taken again to the eye doctor and the power had changed from -3.75 to -0.25. The eye doctor did not understand how it could have happened. He concluded that the previous examinations done by two different were not right.

An 18-year-old had a fatty growth, which looked like a large pea on the outside of the lower left eyelid, that bothered him a lot. He was found to be allergic to the peanut butter sandwiches he ate every day. When he was treated for peanuts, the pea size growth disappeared. From this peanut butter reaction we can formulate a hypothesis that benign or cancerous tumors are often the results of allergies. Finding and treating the causes of the problems can help eliminate growths and tumors.

HEARING LOSS

Food allergies can cause hearing loss. Some children with severe food allergies begin to lose hearing when they are very young. Ear infections, throat infections, runny noses, frequent colds and upper respiratory problems are warning signs in infants and children. When they get ear infections, their pediatricians usually explain to their parents that the canal connecting the throat and the ear is too short in children and food particles easily escape into the ear and cause ear infections. But this explanation is not always true. When the child is allergic to the formula, the food or formula may get into the ear canal and cause the allergic reaction which mimics an infection. If the parent or the pediatrician decides to change the child's food menu to nonallergic items, the child will not have to suffer ear infections or most of the other unwanted childhood diseases.

Such was the case of a two-month old infant, who had a history of vomiting after each meal and chronic constipation. He caught a common cold with a mild fever, a runny nose and an ear infection. The baby was fed with the formula prescribed by the pediatrician and was given antibiotics for 14 days, without any positive results. The child's grandmother visited them during that time. She thought the formula he was drinking was the cause of his health problems. She advised the mother to stop the formula and all the medicines and to feed him with 50 percent low-fat regular homogenized milk. The child's ear, throat, upper-respiratory-tract infection, and low-grade fever cleared up in two days. He also began to have regular bowel movements. This child was not allergic to regular cow's milk, but to all other formulas. Every child may not be as lucky as this one, but if parents and doctors can find some nonallergic formula it will help.

A 4-month-old infant was sick with mild cold symptoms. His pediatrician gave him antibiotic for ten days. He said that the child had an ear infection. But from the time of the second dose of medicine, the infant began crying continuously day and night with out a stop. He cried for three days and two nights, without any sleep or food. He was found to be allergic to the antibiotic. When he was successfully treated for the antibiotic, he stopped crying and began sleeping first time in three days. He was also found to be allergic to the milk he was drinking. That was the cause of the ear infection in the first place.

If the child's food allergy had been allowed to continue untreated or ignored, in time he would have built up more and more allergic reactions and self-damaging toxins. This toxin will affect the energy pathways, neural pathways, organs and related structures. Thus if the target of the toxin is the ear, hearing loss would be the result.

Most people begin to lose hearing in their old age. These are the people who probably fall in the mild to moderate allergy group. They may not show too many allergic manifestations in their young age. The toxin is accumulated from minor allergies and may affect their hearing in old age. If one did not have allergies, hearing loss need not occur just because one is old. Hearing loss due to old age is not a proper diagnosis. Many people with hearing loss who begin to eat the right (non-allergenic) foods experience improved hearing. If the problem is caught in the initial stages, complete recovery is possible. If the damage is less than 20 percent, regeneration of the damaged tissue is possible, and patients can expect a complete cure after successful treatment for all allergies. It might take months or years before they can get good results. If the damage to the tissue is more, then further damage can be prevented with the treatment. Complete reversal may not be possible, but when the patient is under 16, complete reversal is possible most of the time if the problem is allergy related.

Say Good-bye to Illness

A 32-year-old woman suffered from a severe earache and headache on one side since Valentine's Day. She visited her internist and an ear specialist, and took 20 days of antibiotics and pain killers, without any relief. When she came to our office with one of her friends, she was wearing a tiny, single-stone diamond ear ornament which was given to her by her husband for Valentine's Day as a token of his love. She was allergic to the earring top she was wearing. She removed it and put it away and in a few minutes her pain and discomfort disappeared. Eventually, she was treated for the earring top so that she could wear it and please her husband.

Another interesting case of deafness in a young man of eighteen years is noteworthy. He complained of congestion and fullness in his left year for a month. He also suffered from frequent ringing in the ear, light-headedness, and mild to moderate deafness in the left ear. These symptoms all started after last Christmas. He thought he was getting the flu for a few days and did not do anything about it. When the symptoms persisted, he saw a medical internist first, who diagnosed a mild ear infection and prescribed a decongestant and an antibiotic. He tried those and they did not do much good.

Finally, he was sent to our office. When he was evaluated, he was found to be highly allergic to metals. He was wearing a brand new yellow metal wristwatch, and he informed us that it was his girl friend's Christmas gift to him and he has worn it ever since, even to bed. This watch was touching "San Jiao five," one of the main points of the San Jiao acupuncture meridian, which is responsible for the well being of hearing and other related functions. The watch was irritating this point constantly and created a continuous blockage in that meridian, which in turn caused all the above symptoms. Unless treated, the blockages would become larger and finally the related tissues will be damaged. The end result would be complete deafness before too long.

Many times stiffness, pain in the shoulders and upper back tension can be the result of an allergy to jewelry. A 27-year-old female was such a victim of an allergy to gold. She was married at age 22 and, according to her custom, she wore a thick gold chain around her neck all the time. She was not allowed to remove the chain until she died or her husband died. So the tradition goes in India. She began to have severe neck and shoulder pains. She went from doctor to doctor for some relief. One day her pain got so severe, she had to be rushed to the emergency room. X-rays of the neck showed a clean cut of the C5 vertebra exactly beneath where the chain rested. She was kept in the hospital and the vertebra was fused. She was alright for two months. Then she again began to have the excruciating pain all over. This time she came to us, and we found that she was allergic to the thick gold chain she was wearing. She was treated for gold and her neck pains and body aches disappeared. She still wears the chain around her neck. Since her treatment for gold she does not have to worry about the reactions any more.

FIBROMYALGIA

Fibromyalgia syndrome is very frequently allergy related. Fibromyalgia means pain in the muscles, ligaments and tendons. Allergy to whole grains, fruits vegetables, spices and sugar are some of the causes of this disorder seen in our office. Most patients with fibromyalgia say that they ache all over. Their muscles may feel like they have been pulled. Sometimes the muscles twitch and other times they burn. More women than men get this disorder, but it shows up in all ages and sexes.

Symptoms associated with this disorder are deep muscular aching, burning, throbbing, shooting and stabbing. The pain and stiffness are worse in the morning. Fatigue, brain fatigue, sleep disorders, irritable bowel syndrome, migraine headaches, severe premenstrual syndromes, irritable bladder, light-headedness, dry mouth, skin, and eyes are some of the commonly seen problems with fibromyalgia patients.

Since whole grains are harder to digest, it is advisable for these group of people to eat partially processed foods until they eliminate the allergy to the wholesome products.

ALLERGY TO SILICON

Silica silicon dioxide is a chemical compound consisting of silicon and oxygen. Silica occurs widely in rock forming minerals called silicates, which make up much of earth's crust (outside and inside the earth). Some of the items derived from silicates are quartz crystals, ceramics, feldspar, glass, mica, opal, silica gel, silicon and silicone. Many people react to these materials with reactions that vary from person to person. One of the forms of silica is silicone used in implants mainly for cosmetic purposes. If there is an allergy to silicone it can produce various health problems in the person. People can be allergic to silica also. It is used in many products around us such as glasses used on windows, doors, car doors, etc. People who react to silica can get sick riding in a car or sitting near a glass window or door. Silica gel is used as a sealing agent in bathrooms and various other places where there is a leak. It is also used in certain glues.

A 38-year-old woman came in with a history of severe migraines for 20 years. Upon evaluation, it was discovered that

20 years earlier she had silicone implanted to enlarge her breasts. Ever since that time, she had migraines and digestive problems. She was treated for silicone by Nambudripad's Techniques and she got rid of the 20 year old migraine headaches.

Another woman got sick whenever she traveled in her car. She was found to be allergic to the glass doors which was traced to the silica.

SPIDER AND INSECT BITES

Many people react to bites from insects. Spider bites and flea bites are quite fatal at times. Many people react to wasp and bee stings. This case study is taken from another doctor's practice. One of his patients came in with many spider bites on her arms. She was bitten by them while working in her vegetable garden. The bites were very painful and her arms were swollen. The doctor asked her to bring one dead spider from her garden. She was treated by Nambudripad's techniques for allergy to the spider. After successful treatment, her wounds healed, and she was not bothered any more by spider bites from her garden.

Flea bites are another commonly ignored allergic item for many allergic sufferers. A nine year old girl, with a history of severe asthma for eight years, was treated for various allergies and her asthma was under control. She was treated for animal danders; so cats and dogs did not bother her anymore. One day she visited some of her friends, who had a dog, and after a few minutes at her friend's place, her asthma returned. She was allergic to the fleas. When she was treated for the fleas, she stopped having breathing difficulties when near cats and dogs.

MORNING SICKNESS

Morning sickness during pregnancy is due to some kinds of allergies. The mother may be allergic to foods, vitamins (calcium, zinc, salt, sugar, vitamin C, etc.), even to the embryo at times.

A 28-year-old woman was three months pregnant. She vomited frequently and was nauseated almost all the time. She was fed intravenously, since she couldn't keep anything down in her stomach. She was found to be allergic sugar, salt, zinc, vitamin C and vitamin B-complex. When she was treated for all these, she quit vomiting and she did not need intravenous feeding any more.

A 27-year-old woman was four months pregnant with her third child. This time she had continuous cramps in the lower abdomen since the time of conception. Due to pain and discomfort, she could not eat or sleep normally. She lost a lot of weight. She was examined by her gynecologist every week. She placed her on complete bed rest, which made her cramps get worse. Her blood test revealed that she was making antibodies against the baby. Her doctor advised her to have an abortion, since this pregnancy was affecting her health so deeply. She was a true Catholic and she could not even think about any abortion. Kinesiological testing revealed that she was allergic to the fetus. She was treated for the allergy to the fetus with NAET. Less than four hours later her cramps reduced. She had a good night's sleep for the first time in four months. When she woke up next day, she did not have any abdominal cramps and she never did again. A week later her blood was tested and she did not have any antibodies that were previously seen.

Many pregnant women suffer from pre-eclampsia and eclampsia. Women get high blood pressure and their feet and body swell up. Some other symptoms are excessive weight gain, restlessness, sleeplessness, shortness of breath, skin rashes, itching, nausea, light-headedness, unable to urinate freely, etc. Pregnant mothers may be allergic to foods and prenatal vitamins they faithfully take. If the prenatal clinic doctors and assistants were trained to test the allergies kinesiologically for the prenatal vitamins and nutrition, some of these unfortunate incidents could be prevented.

A 39-year-old pregnant woman had sciatic pain for almost a month during her eighth month of pregnancy. Her pain got so severe she had to be confined to bed 24 hours, in spite of all the physical therapy she received. Her husband was a busy cardiologist, who was forced to take time off his busy practice to take care of her. Even with all the tender loving care her pain and discomfort got worse. This was her state when she was brought to our office. Kinesiological testing revealed that she was highly allergic to the prenatal vitamin she was taking so faithfully every day. She was treated for the pill and, less than one hour later, her sciatic pain got relieved never to return.

ALLERGY TO DENTAL ANESTHESIA

A 28-year-old woman had complaints of excruciating pains in her right jaw, along with swelling of the right side of the face, for three weeks. She had some dental work done three weeks ago. She returned to her dentist many times with the same complaint after the initial work. She applied cold and hot compresses according to his advice, took antibiotics and took pain pills. Nothing gave her any relief. When she came to our office, kinesiological testing revealed that she was allergic to the dental anesthetics that was used in the procedure. She was treated for the exact anesthetic with NAET. Her result even amazed the office staff. Half way through the acupuncture treatment, less than 20 minutes, her facial swelling was absolutely gone. At the end of the treatment, she had no pain at all and the pain never returned.

NEWSPAPER INK

Newspaper ink can also cause problems such as backaches, asthma, etc. An example is the case of one particular patient, who had been clear of all asthma symptoms and asthma medication for two years. Then in July 1988, the asthma suddenly recurred, but only in the morning and late evening. Careful elimination of all possible substances linked the occurrence to her reading the newspaper. A call to the printing department at the Orange County Division of the Los Angeles Times newspaper uncovered the fact that they had switched to a new ink during the exact time this patient's asthma returned.

OFFICE PRODUCTS

The office environment is an unexpected culprit of many chronic health problems. Such common place items as fluorescent lighting, computer printer ink, computer keyboards, telephone instruments and paper, which people are in constant daily contact with, have been linked to such problems as fatigue, headaches, shoulder and neck pains, etc. Lead pencils and pens can be a problem due to the allergy to the wood that is used to make pencils. The plastic products used to make pens, markers and highlighters may also cause allergies.

PHARMACY

Many people have allergic reactions to various drugs like antibiotics, analgesics, hormone pills, decongestants, anti-depressants, anti-asthmatics, etc. When one drug does not work or give an allergic reaction, the doctor will prescribe another one. If that also fails to do the job, he or she will try another one until all are run out. Finally, the patient who hoped to get a magical recovery with the drug will lose patience and trust in the efficacy of the pharmaceuticals and even the doctors. The patient's reaction may be so severe, survival from the episode may be doubtful. If the drug was tested for allergy and effectiveness before it was administered, patients, doctors and pharmacists would not have to go through such trying times. Kinesiological testing for allergies and effectiveness should be taught in the school of pharmacy, school of nutrition, school of Western medicine, school of chiropractic medicine, school of dentistry and all other medical schools. Operating room assistants and surgeons should be taught to test the allergy of the surgical materials, transplant materials, organs for transplants, etc. with the patient and make sure the patients are not allergic to them. When the non-allergic materials are used in a procedure chances of reactions and rejection of the transplants are minimal or none. This will give more satisfaction not only to the patients and family but to the treating doctor.

ALLERGY TO CRYSTALS AND STONES

People can be allergic to jewelry and clothing that they are wearing and sometimes to the jewelry and clothes others are wearing. They may also be allergic to items while visiting friends, shopping, attending theaters, going anywhere people congregate. Such was the case of a young woman who was a patient in our office. Whenever she sat in the waiting room, she complained of getting sinus blockages, pain in the upper arms and whole body, and sometimes numbness on certain parts of the body. She claimed that she felt better away from the office. The office staff felt guilty about this and decided to investigate more deeply into this matter.

She was scheduled for treatment, along with another lady who always wore a large crystal pendant, and they were both in the office at the same time waiting for their turn to see the doctor. It was discovered that the first woman was allergic to the crystal that the other woman was wearing. The energy field of crystal was very strong, like diamonds, and this field was affecting the first patient's field from ten feet away. From that day these two patients were scheduled at different times until they were treated for the crystals.

A young man had constant yeast infections, chronic fatigue syndrome, emotional fatigue, night sweats, nervousness, poor memory and various mental disturbances for the last ten years. He had seen a number of medical doctors, chiropractors, acupuncturists, and nutritionists to get some relief. He was also going for psychiatric counseling regularly, since he was often suicidal. He was also treated in our office for over six months for various allergies. He showed marked progress. He stopped having night sweats and fatigue, his memory improved and the yeast infection cleared up for the first time in ten years. He began to live normally, until three or four months later. Then all of a sudden he returned to the office in tears. He said he was almost back to where he started.

We tested him for various items that he was once treated for and found no response in anything whatsoever. Finally we realized that he had lot of jewelry all over him. Four earrings with four different stones in one ear, a heavy necklace with a huge gold and silver pendant, eight rings on the fingers with stones like a star ruby, diamond, emerald, garnet, turquoise, sapphire, etc., and a gold watch studded with diamonds. When he was tested for the stones, he was found to be highly allergic to them. Upon questioning him further, he revealed that he had taken off all the jewelry when he started the treatments with us months ago. He was fond of jewelry and always adorned himself with all these jewels for ten years or so. Now since he was feeling good, he started wearing them again and all the previous symptoms returned. He was treated for all the jewelry and once again he became healthy and happy.

Nambudripad's Allergy Elimination Techniques to treat allergies, and thus eliminate most heath problems, is absolutely a new, revolutionary approach. We must recognize the need for more theoretical work and clinical information. However, there need to be more people who are willing to specialize in this field and make the diagnosis and care of allergic patients their area of specialization within their own fields. The results of patient case histories need to be collected, tabulated, and computerized for satisfactory comparisons. The results of the studies have to be published in the languages of the health care professionals and the patient in charge of his or her own health care. Professionals from different medical fields should be willing to be trained to recognized the symptoms produced by allergens and to relate them to the complex interrelationship between the central nervous system and the biochemical substances and process that occur in us and affect us all.

Until these disorders are fully understood and treatment is made fully available, professionals are encouraged to begin to see their patients in terms of environmental illnesses and to recognize the potential for cure that the holistic techniques of kinesiology, chiropractic and acupuncture offer.

CHAPTER NINETEEN

ALLERGIES AND NUTRITION

Vitamins and trace minerals are essential to life. They contribute to good health by regulating the metabolism and assisting the biochemical processes that release energy from the foods and drinks we consume. Vitamins are micronutrients and the body needs them in small amounts. Even though these are needed in minute amounts, the absence or lack of these essential elements can create various impairments and tissue damages in the body. Water, carbohydrates, fats, proteins and bulk minerals like calcium, magnesium, sodium, potassium and phosphorus are considered to be macronutrients, and we take them into the body via regular food. They are needed in larger amounts. Micro nutrients like vitamins and trace minerals are needed in small amounts in our body. Both, macro and micro nutrients are necessary to produce energy for our daily body functions, as well as growth and development of the body and mind.

Using macronutrients (food & drinks), and micronutrients (vitamins and trace minerals) the body creates some essential chemicals in the body. These are called enzymes and hormones. These are the foundation of human bodily functions. Enzymes are the catalysts or simple activators in the chemical reactions that are continually taking place in the body. Without the appropriate vitamins and trace minerals, the production and function of the enzymes will be incomplete. Prolonged deficiency of the vitamins and minerals can produce immature or incomplete enzyme production, protein synthesis, cell mutation, immature RNA, DNA synthesis, etc., and this can mimic various organic diseases in the body.

Deficiency of the vitamins, and other essentials in the body, can be due to poor intake and poor absorption. Nutritional imbalances are mainly contributed by allergies. When a person's energy field conflicts with nutritional elements like vitamin C, calcium, B-complex, etc., one cannot absorb the essential vitamins and minerals into the body. The body cannot therefore function properly, due to the lack of certain enzymes and mediators, etc., which are supposed to have formed in the presence of these necessary vitamins and minerals. When the body does not produce complete enzymes, hormones and other immune mediators or other body-function mediators, body functions will not proceed as they should. When you do not function properly, and the body malfunctions and continues to malfunction for a while, the temporary dysfunctions can lead to major illnesses.

Vitamin and mineral deficiency syndromes can mimic many other organic diseases in the body. When the body does not function properly, dysfunction will turn into disease; when it starts hurting, patients will seek help. Desperate patients will start visiting any professional health practitioners in search of some relief for their problem. Nutritionists also play a larger role in treating patients. Finally, patients will be placed on large doses of various vitamins and minerals along with health foods.

Many of the patients can have nutritional deficiencies due to poor eating habits. Others may have nutritional deficiencies due to food allergies. People who fall into the category of deficiencies will benefit from the nutritional supplements and megavitamin therapy. The other group, the one with food allergies will not show any improvement. In fact, most of them will get worse on vitamin therapy. People who get well on vitamin therapy will consider megavitamin therapy as a miracle cure, because once they fill up the deficiencies their body functions will restore to normalcy. People who are allergic to vitamins and minerals will get worse on vitamin therapy, because their energy fields repel the energy fields of the vitamins and minerals, so they cannot absorb them. When they eat regular food, a minute amount of vitamins and minerals are circulated through the body. Minute amounts create minute fields and the repulsion is weak. But when one swallows a vitamin or mineral pill, the concentration of the elements is larger than from food items and the repulsion is also larger. This is the reason, very possibly that allergic patients get very sick on vitamin/mineral therapy.

All patients should be tested for possible allergies before they are placed on vitamin therapy. If they are found to be allergic, they should be treated for the allergies before they are supplemented with vitamin and mineral megadoses.

A 34-year-old woman was diagnosed as having chronic fatigue syndrome by a famous doctor and was treated for it. She also suffered from the Epstein-Barr virus and candidiasis and yeast infection. She was treated by him for two years without any relief. Then one of the friends who suffered from a similar complaint had a magical cure with a nutritionist. Hoping to get relief as well, she drove to this nutritionist's office. The cost was a few hundred dollars on her first visit. She was sent home with megadoses of vitamins and mineral supplements, along with the advice to practice good nutrition. She went to a health food store and purchased a lot of health foods. She thought, "This is it" and was whistling, "I am on the way to good health."

Her hopes came crashing down the next day when she woke up with severe body aches and an unbearable headache. She called the doctor, who told her that the toxins are getting out of her system because of change of diet and vitamin/mineral supplements. She waited anxiously for the toxins to get out and leave her body, but her condition got progressively worse. In one week's time, she ended up having bronchitis, a hacking cough, severe joint pains, severe fatigue, headaches, lack of energy, and finally some swelling of the ankles and knees. At this point she quit eating the health foods and vitamins. Her body aches got slightly better; but her respiratory problem persisted. She tried some strong broad spectrum antibiotics for a couple of weeks with no positive results.

She had been suffering from severe bronchitis for six weeks when she came to our office. In the office she was found to be allergic to almost all the foods she was tested for especially, whole wheat, oat bran, bran flakes, etc. She was treated for all the known food allergies first and placed on a diet of nonallergic foods only. In less than two weeks, her bronchitis got better, the cough got better and her energy level picked up. She was on disability when she came to our office. Three and a half months later she went back to work full-time.

Apart from allergies, one needs to know a few things about taking vitamins and minerals. Of the major vitamins, few are water soluble and few are fat soluble. Water soluble vitamins are vitamin C and the B-complex vitamins. Fat soluble vitamins are vitamins A,D,E, and K. It is believed that water soluble vitamins must be taken into the body daily, as they can not be stored, and are excreted within one to four days, even though our clinical experience has proven this is not true all the time.

Many times when a patient is allergic to vitamin B-complex, she or he can not digest grains. When one can not digest grains, she or he will have B-complex deficiencies. When one gets treated for allergies via NAET, she/he can eat grains without any ill effect. When she/he begins to eat grains, she/he will begin to assimilate B-complex vitamins. Through kinesiological testing, we have seen large deficiencies of B-vitamins. In some cases, we have seen B-complex deficiency amounting to fifteen thousand to twenty thousand times normal daily recommended allowances. After supplementing with large amounts of B-complex for a few weeks (20-30 times of RDA amount per day), the deficiency was reduced to zero requirement level. We have done this experiment over and over in hundreds of patients. After supplementing for weeks we have been able to remove the vitamin B-complex deficiency symptoms completely. This proves that vitamin B-complex is stored in the body. This experiment was done on vitamin C also, and we have received similar results. More research is needed on a larger number of patients in this area to verify these findings.

Oil soluble or fat soluble vitamins are stored for longer periods of time in the body's fatty tissue and the liver. When one is allergic to fat soluble vitamins, they begin to store abnormally in the body in unwanted places. Some of these abnormal storages of these vitamins can be seen as lipomas, warts, skin tags, benign tumors inside or outside the body, etc.

Taking vitamins and minerals in their proper balance is important to the proper functioning of all vitamins. Excess consumption of an isolated vitamin or mineral can produce unpleasant deficiency symptoms of that particular nutrient. High doses of one element can also cause depletion of other nutrients in the body, causing other problems. Most of these vitamins work synergetically, complimenting each other's function or strengthening each other's function.

Vitamins and minerals should be taken with meals unless specified otherwise. Oil-soluble vitamins should be taken before meals, and water soluble vitamins should be taken between or after meals. But when one is taking megadoses of any of these, they should always be taken with or after meals. Vitamins and minerals, as nutritional supplements taken with meals, will supply the missing nutrients in our daily diets that may be deficient in appropriate nutritional elements.

Synthetic vitamins are produced in a laboratory from isolated chemicals with similar quality of natural vitamins. Although there are no major chemical differences between a vitamin found in food and one created in a laboratory, natural supplements do not contain other unnatural ingredients. Supplements that are not labeled natural may include coal tars, artificial coloring, preservatives, sugars, starches, as well as other additives. Natural vitamin bottles may contain vitamins that have not been extracted from a natural food source.

There are various books available on nutrition today that are helpful to understand about vitamins and their assimilative processes, if any one wants to further one's knowledge in nutrition. Some of the of books are listed at the end of this book in the bibliography section.

VITAMIN A

Clinical studies have proved vitamin A and beta-carotene as very powerful immuno-stimulants and protective agents. Vitamin A is essential for a variety of normal body functions. It's deficiency can cause disturbed lymphocyte production and function. A decreased lymphocyte production, or abnormal lymphocyte production, can cause decreased phagocyte activity which may lead to lower immune functioning and auto immune functioning.

Vitamin A is necessary for proper vision, prevents night blindness, skin disorders, acne, protects against colds, influenza and other infections. It enhances immunity, helps heal ulcers and wounds and helps in maintenance of epithelial cell tissue. It is necessary for the growth of bones and teeth. Vitamin A is an antioxidant and helps to protect the cells against cancer and other diseases. Beta-carotene, from the vegetable source, converts into vitamin A in the liver, which is very good for cancer prevention. Vitamin A helps in protein assimilation. This also helps to slow the aging process. This helps to build body resistance, fight respiratory infections, promote growth, maintain clear, healthy skin, hair, nails, teeth and gums.

When one is allergic to vitamin A, or when vitamin A does not absorb normally in the body, skin tags, warts blemishes, etc. appear on the skin surface. It is a wonder vitamin. If there is a problem with proper absorption and utilization of vitamin A in one's body, one can experience toxic symptoms, such as poor or blurry vision, repeated respiratory infection, lowered immunity, skin problems like rashes, boils, acne, unhealthy, wrinkled skin, premature aging, loss of hair and nails, unhealthy teeth and gums, headaches of various nature, infertility, irregular menses, pain in the joints, gastrointestinal disturbances like nausea, vomiting, diarrhea, indigestion, etc. If the allergy is treated, and if diet is properly supplemented, the toxic symptoms can be completely eliminated.

Vitamin A works best with B-complex, vitamin D, vitamin E, calcium, phosphorus and zinc. Zinc is needed to get vitamin A out of the liver, where it is usually stored in the body. Large doses of vitamin A should be taken only under proper supervision, otherwise it can accumulate in the body and become toxic.

Food sources of vitamin A are fish liver oil, milk and diary products, butter, egg yolks, corn, green leafy or yellow vegetables, yellow fruits, liver, alfalfa, apricots, asparagus, beets, broccoli, carrots, swiss chard, dandelion greens, garlic, kale, mustard, papayas, parsley, peaches, red peppers, sweet potatoes, spinach, spirulina, pumpkin, yellow squash, turnip greens and watercress.

A seven year old boy had a great many problems with vision. He was tested by two ophthalmologists at two different locations and given high-powered eye glasses. Then he was treated by NAET for allergy to vitamin A and given large doses of vitamin A (100,000 units daily), as a supplement for one month. Then he was tested again for his vision. His eyeglass power was down by 50 percent. After six months of supplementation, he was tested again and his prescription power was down even further to minimal numbers. He was given 50,000 units of vitamin A for another six months, then 25,000 units for one more year. Now, two years later he doesn't need glasses at all; he can see and function well without glasses.

Many teenagers with allergy to vitamin A get acne, blemishes and other skin problems. Many people with allergy to vitamin A develop skin tags, and warts, pimples, around the neck, arms, etc. It is also one of the causes of premenstrual syndrome. When they get treated and properly supplemented with vitamin A, the skin clears up and PMS problems become less severe.

Vitamin deficiencies can be one of the problems of infertility, since the integrity of the endometrium depends on vitamin A assimilation. Vitamin A helps too form the healthy mucous membrane. A 34 year old female was trying to get pregnant for years, without any success. She was found to be highly allergic to vitamin A and essential fatty acids. After she was treated for these items, she was placed on tankuei and peony formula (a chinese herbal formula for regulating the hormonal functions in women, thus helps with infertility). Within four months she became pregnant.

It is also necessary to prevent aging. A 73-year-old woman, with a lot of wrinkles, was treated for vitamin A and supplemented with 75,000 IU of vitamin A daily for three months. Her wrinkles began to subside gradually. Whenever she went off vitamin A supplementation for a couple of weeks, her wrinkles would begin to return. When she realized this, she continued to take vitamin A somewhere in the range of 25,000 to 50,000 IU daily. This kept her skin younger and smoother without very many wrinkles.

A young girl used to get repeated upper respiratory infections. She was found to be highly allergic to vitamin A. She was treated for vitamin A and supplemented regularly with vitamin A. Within a few months, she built up enough resistance and did not get frequent upper respiratory infections any more.

A 54-year-old female with lots of warts and pimples around the neck and near the hairline was allergic to vitamin A. After she was treated with NAET for vitamin A, she was supplemented with 50,000 units for six months. Her skin cleared completely.

A 48-year-old male had a history of periodic bleeding from the rectum for six years. His everyday diet included lots of raw and cooked carrots and cantaloupes. He was treated for vitamin A and beta-carotene using NAET. This put an end to his six year old problem.

VITAMIN D

Vitamin D is often called the sunshine vitamin. It is a fat-soluble vitamin, acquired through sunlight or food sources. Ultraviolet rays act on the oils of the skin to produce the vitamin, which is then absorbed into the body. Vitamin D is absorbed from foods when eaten through the intestinal wall. Smog reduces the vitamin D producing rays of the sun. Dark-skinned people and sun tanned people do not absorb vitamin D from the sun. Vitamin D helps to utilize calcium and phosphorus in the human body. It is important in the prevention and treatment of osteoporosis. It helps to improve the body's resistance against respiratory tract infections, helps to assimilate vitamin A and keeps skin and bones healthy. When there is an allergy to vitamin D, the vitamin is not absorbed into the body through foods or from the sun.

People with an allergy to vitamin D can show deficiency syndromes such as rickets, severe tooth decay, softening of teeth and bones, osteomalacia, senile osteoporosis, sores on the skin, blisters on the skin while walking in the sun, severe sunburns when exposed to the sun, etc. Sometimes allergic persons can show toxic symptoms if they take vitamin D without clearing its allergy. These symptoms include mental confusion, unusual thirst, sore eyes, itching skin, vomiting, diarrhea, urinary urgency, calcium deposits in the blood vessels and bones, restlessness in the sun, and inability to bear heat. Vitamin D works best with vitamin A, vitamin C, choline, calcium and phosphorus.

Food sources of vitamin D are fish-liver oils, dairy products fortified with vitamin D, alfalfa, butter, egg yolk, liver, sunshine, milk and milk products, meat, fish, eggs, cereal products, sweet potatoes, vegetable oils, beans, fruits and vegetables.

When an allergy to vitamin D is treated by Nambudripad's Techniques, the deficiency or toxic symptoms can be eliminated and, gradually with the proper supplementation, normal health can be obtained.

A 30-year-old male complained of restlessness when he was in the sun. He also complained of canker sores in the mouth, if he walked in the sun. He was found to be highly allergic to vitamins A, C, D and calcium. He was treated for vitamins A, C and calcium. His symptoms were reduced dramatically, but he still had them. Finally, when he was treated for vitamin D, he began to feel comfortable under the sun. He also stopped having canker sores in the mouth.

A teenager who had severe acne on her face was found to be allergic to vitamin D but not vitamin A. Whenever she took supplemental vitamins A and D, she began having more acne.

Whenever she took only vitamin A and avoided dairy products and fish, her skin became better. When she was treated for vitamin D, she could eat milk products and fish without causing any skin problems.

VITAMIN E

Vitamin E is an antioxidant that prevents cancer and cardiovascular disease. The body needs zinc in order to maintain the proper levels of vitamin E in thee blood. Vitamin E is a fat-soluble vitamin and is stored in the liver, fatty tissues, heart, muscles, testes, uterus, blood, adrenal glands and pituitary glands. Vitamin E is excreted in the feces if too much is taken. Even though it is fat soluble, it is stored for a short period of time in the body.

Among Vitamin E's numerous functions is its ability to suppress cellular aging due to oxidation. Vitamin E improves circulation, repairs tissue, treats fibrocystic breasts and premenstrual syndrome. It also promotes normal clotting and healing. It reduces scarring and blood pressure, helps prevent cataracts, leg cramps, age spots or liver spots. It is an antioxidant, and it protects the lungs against air pollution and thus supplies more oxygen to the body. It can help prevent or dissolve blood clots, because it has an anticoagulant property. It promotes healing of minor wounds and skin irritation and can prevent scarring if applied locally. It has a big role in fertility. Vitamins E and A help the uterus to prepare for pregnancy. Vitamin E aids in prevention of miscarriages, alleviates fatigue and helps to strengthen tired lower limbs after long walks or exercise. It also helps to reduce leg cramps by its vasodilating action. It also acts as a diuretic.

Deficiency syndromes include destruction of red blood cells, muscle degeneration, some anemia, infertility, heart and circulation problems. If one is allergic to vitamin E he can show all the deficiency syndromes. After the proper elimination of vitamin E allergy, it can be supplemented to get positive benefits.

Vitamin E is found in the following food sources: vegetable oils, whole grains, dark green leafy vegetables, nuts, seeds, legumes, dry beans, brown rice, cornmeal, eggs, desiccated liver, milk, oatmeal, organ meats, sweet potatoes, wheat germ, broccoli, brussels sprouts, leafy greens, spinach, enriched flour and whole wheat.

A 38-year-old female had a scaly, dry skin on the arms and legs. She tried many different creams, including cortisone creams. Dry skin peeled periodically and was quite rough, causing pain and a burning sensation all the time. When she came to us, she was tested on various items for allergies and found to be highly allergic to vitamin E. She was using many creams, soaps and shampoos, which contained large amounts of vitamin E. She also took 400 IU of vitamin E daily as a supplement. After she was treated for vitamin E by Nambudripad's Techniques, her skin became smoother and softer. She now uses the vitamin E cream effectively.

A woman came to our office with a swollen, infected, crusty, weeping area where she had her ear pierced. She said that she had this problem for a few years now. She had seen other doctors, including dermatologists and had used a few creams including cortisone creams. If she did not wear any earring the problem area began to heal. As soon as she started wearing any type of earring, the problem returned. She was asked to bring all her earrings. When she was tested for them she was found to be allergic to the earrings or its posts. While testing one of the earrings, it was found to be sticky and oily. When she was questioned about that she said that she used a cream to lubricate the post before she inserted it into the ear lobe. This was a highly concentrated vitamin E cream. On allergy testing she was found to be highly allergic to vitamin E. After treatment for the allergy by Nambudripad's Allergy Elimination Techniques, and stoppage of the use of any cream to lubricate the ear, she hasn't had the problem.

VITAMIN K

Vitamin K is needed for blood clotting. It is also needed in the formation of bones. Vitamin K is necessary to convert glucose into glycogen for storage in the liver. Vitamin K is a fat-soluble vitamin, very essential to the formation of prothrombin, a blood-clotting material. It helps in the blood-clotting mechanism, prevents hemorrhages like nosebleeds and intestinal bleeding, and helps to reduce excessive menstrual flow.

An allergy to vitamin K can produce deficiency syndromes such as prolonged bleeding time, intestinal diseases like sprue, etc., and colitis.

Vitamin K is found in alfalfa, broccoli, dark green leafy vegetables, soy beans, black strap molasses, brussels sprouts, cabbage, cauliflower, egg yolks, liver, oatmeal, oats, rye, safflower oil and wheat.

As said earlier, allergy to vitamin K can cause blood clotting disorders. A four year old boy was suffering from hemophilia since he was two years old. He bruised in the various joints frequently, especially if he walked fast, ran or played with other kids in the school. Whenever he received an attack, he had to stay home with ice compresses on the affected joints for the next few days. He was found to be allergic to cabbage, which was one of his staple diets in the house. When he was treated for cabbage and vitamin K by NAET, his hemophilia like symptoms disappeared. His family doctor declared him to be under remission for hemophilia. He is an active 3rd grader now, with out any trace of his previous symptoms.

A 38-year-old woman came in with a complaint of severe uterine bleeding for six weeks. She was one of our pioneer patients, who previously had received treatment for various allergies. She had consulted a gynecologist and the doctor could not find any reason for the sudden bleeding. When she came to our office, it was discovered from her history that one of the nutritionists had placed her on various vitamin and mineral supplements about six weeks previously. One of them was 15 alfalfa tables twice a day. She was found to be allergic to alfalfa and vitamin K. She was treated for vitamin K and her bleeding stopped within six to eight hours after the successful treatment.

Another 28-year-old girl complained of severe PMS and cramps during her periods. She also observed that if she ate salads with alfalfa sprouts her PMS was worse. She was found to be highly allergic to vitamin K, alfalfa and cabbage. Her PMS dramatically diminished after treatments for vitamin K.

A 42-year-old man had a unique problem. He passed and sprayed fresh blood whenever he defecated; he had no hemorrhoids and had no cramps or pains. He felt lethargic and fatigued all the time. His history revealed that he had given up eating red meats, for health reasons, and was eating mostly vegetables, salads, fruits and whole grains. He was found to be allergic to vitamins C and K, which were in all the vegetables and fruits he ate. After he was treated for vitamins C and K by Nambudripad's Techniques he hasn't had the above-mentioned problems in six years.

VITAMIN B

Approximately 15 vitamins make up the B-complex family. Each one of them has unique, very important functions in one's body. If the body does not absorb and utilize any or all of the B-vitamins, various health problems can result. B-complex vitamins are very essential for emotional, physical and physiological well being of the human body. It is a nerve food, so it is necessary for the proper growth and maintenance of the nervous system and brain function. It also keeps the nerves well fed so that nerves are kept calm and the person maintains a good mental attitude. Certain B vitamins function as enzyme precursors and aids in digestion. Among the B vitamins and their function are:

B1 - This vitamin has a great effect on the nervous system and mental attitude and aids in digestion of sugar and carbohydrates and helps to treat alcoholics. It also reduces stress by calming the nerves.

B2 - Aids in growth and reproduction. Promotes healthy skin, nails and hair, aids in digestion of carbohydrates, fats and proteins.

B6 - Aids in digestion and assimilation of proteins and fats. Prevents various nervous and skin disorders; reduces morning sickness and nausea in general. Promotes synthesis of nucleic acids, reduces neuralgia and neuritis by calming the nerves. Works as a natural diuretic.

B12 - Prevents anemia, regenerates red blood cells, increases overall energy, maintains a healthy nervous system, aids in digestion of carbohydrates, fats and proteins, improves concentration, memory and emotional balance.

FOLIC ACID

Essential to the formation of red blood cells and to prevent anemia, aids in protein metabolism, aids in production of nucleic acids, helps in cell division, essential for utilization of sugar and amino acids, improves lactation, delays hair graying when used with paba and pantothenic acid.

INOSITOL

Promotes healthy hair and prevents hair loss, aids in redistribution of body fat, lowers cholesterol and also produces a calming effect. Inositol, choline, pantothenic acid and B-12 taken together help improve concentration and memory.

For more information on particular vitamins, their functions and deficiency syndromes, refer to the appropriate reference in the bibliography.

If one is allergic to any B-vitamin, allergic symptoms can appear in many forms. The doctor has to take special care to isolate the allergic vitamin and treat to alleviate the problem. B-vitamins are seen in almost all foods we eat. Some of them are destroyed by cooking and heating, but some are not destroyed by processing or preparation. People who are allergic to B-vitamins can get mild to severe reactions just by eating the foods alone. If they are supplemented with vitamin B-complex, without being aware of the allergies, such people can get exaggerated reactions. One has to be very cautious while taking B-complex commonly known as stress vitamins.

Food sources of B vitamins include whole grains, seeds, legumes, milk products, pork, liver, beef, green leafy vegetables, potatoes, nuts, eggs, fish, root vegetables, green vegetables, fruits, brewer's yeast, brans and wheat germ.

Dr. Carlton Frederic in his book, *Psychonutrition*, tried to point out that nutritional deficiencies are the causes of most of the mental sicknesses in psychiatric facilities. He tried to prove his theory by giving large doses of vitamin B-complex, especially B-12, to some of the psychiatric patients. Fifty percent of the patients got better, were cured of their mental sickness and went back to live normal lives. But another 50 percent got worse and made minerals.

A few minerals are extremely essential for our daily functions. While other metals and trace minerals are mentioned here, for more information on other minerals, please refer to the appropriate references in the bibliography.

CALCIUM

Calcium is one of the essential minerals in the body. Calcium works with phosphorus, magnesium, iron, vitamins A, C and D. Calcium helps to maintain strong bones and healthy teeth. It regulates the heart functions and helps to relax the nerves and muscles. It induces relaxation and sleep.

Deficiencies in calcium result in rickets, osteomalacia, osteoporosis, hyperactivity, restlessness, inability to relax, generalized aches and pains, joint pains, formation of bone spurs, backaches, PMS, cramps in the legs and heavy menstrual flow.

Calcium food sources are mild products, soybean, sardine, oyster, salmon, nuts, dried beans and green leafy vegetables. If someone is allergic to calcium, he can get deficiency syndromes in exaggerated forms whenever he eats foods containing calcium. When the allergy is eliminated by Nambudripad's Allergy Elimination Techniques, he can be supplemented appropriately to get maximum health benefits.

Many asthmatic people, with upper respiratory problems, respond well to calcium supplementation. Many people with abdominal pains, dysentery, insomnia, skin problems, nervousness, dyslexia, canker sores, post-nasal drip, hyperactivity, obesity, and arthritis respond well to allergy treatments for calcium and later supplementation. Many women who have heavy menstrual flow respond well to allergy treatment for calcium and later supplementation. When people are on cortisone treatment they need to take more calcium.

A 26-year-old female complained of heart palpitations whenever she consumed milk or milk products. She was found to be allergic to calcium. When she was treated by Nambudripad's Techniques for calcium, she stopped having heart palpitations when she ate milk products.

A 14-year-old boy complained of severe leg cramps and extreme tiredness after baseball practice. His parents complained that he was not growing tall enough for his age. One of the nutritionists advised him to take calcium supplements. He go very sick with severe joint pains and was found to be allergic to calcium. After he was treated for calcium by Nambudripad's Techniques, his cramps and joint pains got better. When he was supplemented with calcium, not only did he get stronger, he began to grow taller. He grew six inches in a few months.

A 53-year-old female had severe skin rashes and blisters, which eventually turned into ulcers. She bruised easily and had black and blue marks all over the body. She said that she started drinking more milk and taking calcium supplements to prevent osteoporosis. She was found to be allergic to milk products and calcium. When she was treated for them, her skin problems cleared up.

A 42-year-old female complained of severe backache. She took calcium pills which made it worse. She was not allergic to calcium, but she was allergic to the binders used to make the pills. When she was treated for the binders of the calcium pills, she stopped having the backaches. When she took calcium pills after treatment she felt more relaxed.

A five year old boy was very hyperactive. He got very restless and noisy soon after he drank milk. He was allergic to milk and calmed down greatly, after he was treated for milk and calcium.

A 36-year-old female complained of severe uterine bleeding, with heavy clots during her menstrual periods, which lasted for almost ten days each time. She had various treatments, including hormone shots, prior to coming to our office. She was found to be allergic to calcium. She was treated for allergy to calcium by Nambudripad's Allergy Elimination Techniques and supplemented with large quantities (4,000 to 6,000 mg) of calcium daily. Her periods became regular and flow became normal within two months.

A 52-year-old male had five different surgeries on his left knee for pain. He was scheduled for the sixth surgery when he was seen in our office. He was a printer by profession and had to stand on his feet the whole day. He was found to be very deficient in calcium. He was not allergic to calcium. He was on fad diets to fight his mild obesity. He was 20 pounds overweight. This hard working man did not get enough calcium from his food intake to meet his daily needs. He was supplemented with 6,000 mg. of calcium daily for one month. He stopped having knee pains. Three years later he still remains pain-free.

Iron is one of the essential minerals, necessary for the production hemoglobin (red blood corpuscles), myoglobin (red pigment in muscles), and certain enzymes. In one month, women lose more iron than men. Iron requires copper, cobalt, manganese, and vitamin C for proper assimilation. Iron is also necessary for proper metabolization of B vitamins. Iron aids in growth, promotes resistance to disease, prevents fatigue, prevents and cures iron deficiency anemia.

Food sources for iron include apricots, peaches, bananas, black molasses, prunes, raisins, brewer's yeast, whole grain cereals, spinach, beets, alfalfa, sunflower seeds, walnuts, sesame seeds, dried beans, lentils, liver, egg yolk, red meats, pork, kidney, heart, clams, oysters, oatmeal and asparagus.

IRON

Iron deficiency results in anemia. People with allergy to iron do not absorb iron from food. They suffer from iron deficiency anemia, even though they take iron supplements. A person with iron allergy can get various problems from iron supplementation or eating iron-containing foods.

A 32-year-old male complained of backaches since he was a teenager. On certain days his backache was very severe, and he had to stay home in bed for three to four days at a time. He could not hold a permanent job and worked on a daily basis through a temporary agency. He had undergone various diagnostic tests for his backache, but no cause was found. In our office, this man was found to be highly allergic to all the foods containing iron. When he was treated for iron by Nambudripad's Techniques, he began to feel great relief from his chronic backache. Incidently, he took 18 consecutive treatments to get desensitized for iron. This young man does not get severe backaches anymore. He was able to work full-time without getting sick for the past one and half years.

CHROMIUM

Chromium is an essential element to metabolize sugar, to treat diabetes, to treat hypoglycemia and to treat alcoholism. A deficiency results in arteriosclerosis, hypoglycemia and diabetes.

Food sources include whole grain cereals, wheat germ, corn oil, brewers' yeast, mushroom, liver, raw sugar, red meat, shell fish, chicken and clams.

COBALT

Cobalt is essential for red blood cells, since it is part of vitamin B-12. Deficiency results in B-12 deficiency anemia.

Food sources are all green leafy vegetables, meat, liver, kidney, figs, buckwheat, oysters, clams and milk.

COPPER

Copper is required to convert the body's iron into hemoglobin. Combined with the amino acid thyroxin, it helps to produce the pigment factor for hair and skin. It is essential for utilization of vitamin C. Deficiency results in anemia and edema. Toxicity symptoms are insomnia, hair loss, irregular menses and depression.

Food sources of copper are almonds, beans, peas, green leafy vegetables, whole grain products, prunes, raisins, liver, dried beans, whole wheat, beef, most seafood and copper piping water supply.

FLUORINE

Sodium fluoride is added to drinking water. Calcium fluoride is seen in natural food sources. Fluorine decreases chances of dental carries, too much can discolor teeth. It also strengthens the bones. Deficiency leads to tooth decay. Toxicity or allergy symptoms include dizziness, nausea, poor appetite, skin rashes, itching, yeast infections, mental confusion, muscle spasms, mental fogginess and arthritis. Treatment for fluoride will eliminate possible allergies.

Food sources include fluoridated drinking water, seafood, gelatin, sunflower seeds, milk products, carrots, garlic, green leafy vegetable and almonds.

IODINE

Two thirds of the body's iodine is in the body's thyroid gland. Since the thyroid gland controls metabolism, and iodine influences the thyroid, an undersupply of this mineral can result in weight gain, general fatigue and slow mental reaction. Iodine helps to keep the body thin, promotes growth, gives more energy, improves mental alertness, promotes the growth of hair, nails and teeth.

A deficiency in iodine can cause overweight, hyperthyroidism, goiters and lack of energy. Among its food sources are kelp, seafood, iodized salt, vegetables grown in iodine-rich soil and onion.

MAGNESIUM

Magnesium is necessary for the metabolism of calcium, vitamin C, phosphorus, sodium, potassium and vitamin A. It is essential for the normal functioning of nerves and muscles. It also helps convert blood sugar into energy. It works as a natural tranquilizer, milk laxative and diuretic. Diuretics deplete magnesium. Alcoholics and asthmatics are deficient in magnesium.

Food sources of magnesium include nuts, soybeans, raw and cooked green leafy vegetables, almonds, whole grains, sunflower seeds, brown rice and sesame seeds.

Manganese helps to activate digestive enzymes in the body. It is important in the formation of thyroxine, the principal hormone of the thyroid gland. It is necessary for the proper digestion and utilization of food. Manganese is important in reproduction and the normal functioning of the central nervous system. It helps to eliminate fatigue, improves memory, reduces nervous irritability and relaxes the mind. A deficiency may result in recurrent attacks of dizziness and poor memory.

Food sources include green leafy vegetables, spinach, beets, Brussels sprouts, blueberries, oranges, grapefruits, apricots, the outer coating of nuts and grains (bran), peas, kelp, egg yolks, wheat germ and nuts.

MOLYBDENUM

Molybdenum helps in carbohydrate and fat metabolism. It is a vital part of the enzyme responsible for iron utilization. Among its food sources are whole grains, brown rice, brewer's yeast, legumes, buckwheat, millet and dark green leafy vegetables.

PHOSPHORUS

Phosphorus is involved in virtually all physiological chemical reactions in the body. It is necessary for normal bone and teeth formation. It is important for heart regularity, and is essential for normal kidney function. It provides energy and vigor by helping in the fat and carbohydrate metabolism. It promotes growth and repairs in the body. It is essential for healthy gums and teeth. Vitamin D and calcium are essential for its proper functioning.

Food sources of phosphorus are whole grains, seeds, nuts, legumes, milk products, egg, fish, corn, dried fruits, poultry and meat.

POTASSIUM

Potassium works with sodium to regulate the body's water balance and to regulate the heart rhythm. It helps in clear thinking by sending oxygen to the brain. A deficiency in potassium results in edema, hypoglycemia, nervous irritability, and muscle weakness.

Among its food sources are all vegetables, especially green leafy vegetables, oranges, whole grains, sunflower seeds, nuts, bananas, potatoes, potato peelings, citrus fruits, melons, tomatoes, watercress and mint.

SELENIUM

Selenium is an antioxidant. It works with vitamin E, slowing down the aging process, prevents hardening of tissues and helps to retain youthful appearance. Selenium is also known to alleviate hot flashes and menopausal distress. It prevents dandruff. Some researches have found selenium to neutralize certain carcinogens and provide protection from some cancers.

Food sources include brewer's yeast, wheat germ, sea water, kelp, garlic, mushrooms, seafood, milk, eggs, whole grains, beef, fish, beans, most vegetables, bran, tuna fish, onions, tomatoes and broccoli.

SODIUM

Sodium is essential for normal growth and normal body functioning. It works with potassium to maintain the sodium-potassium pump in the body. Potassium is found inside the cells and sodium is found outside. It is essential to maintain processed foods including most fast foods. Food sources are salt, shell fish, carrots, beets, artichokes, beef, brain, kidney and bacon.

SULPHUR

Sulphur is essential for healthy hair, skin and nails. It helps maintain the oxygen balance necessary for proper brain function. It works with B-complex vitamins for basic body metabolism. It is a part of tissue building amino acid. It tones up the skin and makes the hair lustrous and helps fight bacterial infection. Among its food sources are radishes, turnips, onions, celery, string beans, watercress, soybean, fish, meat, lean beef, dried beans, eggs, cabbage, grapes, raisins, dried foods, wines, alcoholic beverages, saccharin, Sweet and Low, sulfites and sulfates.

VANADIUM

Vanadium prevents heart attacks. It inhibits the formation of cholesterol in blood vessels. Its food sources include fish.

ZINC

Zinc is essential to form certain enzymes and hormones in the body. It is very necessary for protein synthesis. It is important for blood stability and in maintaining the body's acid-alkaline balance. It is important in the development of reproductive organs and helps to normalize the prostate glands in males. It helps in treatment of mental disorders and speeds up healing of wounds and cuts on the body. Zinc helps with the growth of fingernails and eliminates cholesterol deposits in the blood vessels.

Food sources of zinc include wheat bran, wheat germ, pumpkin seeds, sunflower seeds, brewers' yeast, milk, eggs, onions, green leafy vegetables, oysters, herrings, peas, brown rice, fish, mushrooms, lamb, beef, pork, nonfat dry milk and mustard.

TRACE MINERALS

Even though trace minerals are needed in our body, they are seen in trace amounts only. Definite functions of the trace minerals are not known to the researchers but deficiencies can definitely contribute toward health problems. Its food sources include alfalfa, kelp, seafood and sea water.

AMINO ACIDS

All proteins are made up of amino acids. They are the building blocks of protein. There are 22 different types of amino acids. Some can be made in the body and are called non essential amino acids. Eight are not produced in the body and are known as essential amino acids. These essential amino acids have to be absorbed from food. The eight essential amino acids are lysine, methionine, leucine, threonine, valine, tryptophan, isoleucine and phenylalanine. Children also need histidine and arginine.

Food sources for essential amino acids are meat, fish, poultry and dairy products, which are complete protein foods. Most vegetables, grains and fruits are incomplete proteins.

From some of the case histories, the reader may gain an understanding of the importance of good nutrition (non-allergic nutrients) in one's life to maintain a proper balance of the body's functions. The body needs all the essential vitamins and minerals in proper proportion for its normal function. If there is any deficiency of the vitamins, minerals, trace minerals, or amino acids, it can be seen as some functional disorder or other problem. If it can be found in time and treated or supplemented with appropriate amounts, many unnecessary discomforts can be avoided.

LECITHIN

Lecithin is needed by every living cell in the human body. Cell membranes, which regulate which nutrients may leave or enter the cell, are largely composed of lecithin. Cell membranes would harden with out lecithin. Its structure protects the cells from damage by oxidation. The protective sheaths surrounding the brain are composed of lecithin, and the muscles and nerve cells also contain this essential fatty substance. Lecithin is composed of choline, inositol and linoleic acids. It acts as an emulsifying agent.

It helps prevent arteriosclerosis, protects against cardiovascular disease, increase brain function, and promotes energy. It helps the fat to digest better and helps the cholesterol to be dispersed in water and removed from the body. The vital organs and arteries are protected from fatty build-up with the inclusion of lecithin in the diet. Most lecithin is derived from soybean, eggs, brewer's yeast, grains, legumes, fish and wheat germ.

CHAPTER TWENTY

TESTIMONIALS FROM THE PROFESSIONALS

Having been into preventive health care for 30 years, there isn't any method that I have seen that can surpass NAET. It is a profound and fascinating technique of correcting allergies, which is an underlying cause of most health problems and disease.

Marie Gold, ND, RMT
921 Oakland Avenue
Indiana, Pennsylvania 15701

We, at the Three Vital Treasures Acucenter, have been using Nambudripad's Technique to treat allergic conditions for about a year. This approach is a welcome adjunct to traditional Chinese Medicine. I am most pleased with the results!

Alexander Horvath, B.S., L.Ac.
California

I have been studying with Dr. Devi Nambudripad, using her technique for a year. In working with patients for the past 25 years as an R.N., and eight years as a Doctor of Oriental Medicine, I have come to similar conclusions regarding allergic conditions as being the root of a vast number of diseases. I am excited to discover an approach to this pervasive health problem that is effective, non-invasive and practical.

Bonnie McLean, L.Ac., O.M.D., R.N.
Topanga, California

I would like to share with you some of my success with NAET treatments. The first case is a 24-year-old, white lady who suffered from severe bronchial asthma. Now, after 14 treatments, she is free of asthmatic attacks and does not have to use too many drugs.

The second case is a 50-year-old lady, who had itching all over the body, for some time. She had been examined and treated with traditional allergists and by many skin specialists without much improvement. After 15 treatments, she has been free of itching and skin problems for the last five months.

Another 35-year-old, white male suffered from juvenile diabetes. He lost the ability to smell. After 12 treatments, he got his sense of smell back. His insulin requirements are steadily going down.

Another old male patient, who had cancer in the colon, was suffering from pain in the stomach. He was on chemotherapy and was given strong pain killers and tranquilizers, but he received no relief from the pain. After using NAET for the chemotherapy agents, he got relief from the pain. After three more treatments, his manifestations of cancer have decreased immensely.

I want to thank you again for treating my daughter, Adi, for her allergies. She is a very healthy and happy six-year old now. I have used this method successfully on hundreds of allergic patients and they all have been able to resume a normal life!

Dr. Samuel Hendler, M.D.
Ear, Nose and Throat Specialist
Medical 18, Rains St.,
Tel-Aviv 64381
Tel. 03-235792

We, Jim and George, owe Dr. Devi S. Nambudripad, a rejuvenation, a keen and heightened sense of well being, a more refined sense of taste and enjoyment of food, as we are rid our allergies for different substances, thanks to her acupuncture treatments. This testimony may be misleading, as it may seem exclusively to stress the effectiveness the treatment. The treatment has been healing, because Dr. Devi, herself a victim of food allergies for years, explored the medical field for self healing, when one or the other systems proved futile to restore her to normal health and finally discovered her freedom from an allergy in her own method of treatment. This genius of an Indian lady first applied techniques to herself and her family members that later proved to be deliverance from various afflictions for hundreds of patients, drawn from a wide spectrum of society.

Scientific credibility is based on results, repeated and replicative. To that end, we herewith contribute our own testimonial. As a professional dealing with other professionals in divergent fields, Dr. Devi could sense and appreciate the needs of other inquiring minds to know the scientific basis of her treatment and completely satisfy our need to understand. This pedagogy helped us to go through whatever was required, as a result, a fuller life has been the boon. We owe Dr. Devi not only healing, but gratitude and admiration.

Fr. James Williams, M.S.
    and
Fr. George Murickam, S.J.
La Mirada, California

I always considered myself an open-minded physician, but must admit, I attended Dr. Devi's course with great skepticism. After all, who would believe that a simple 15 minute treatment utilizing acupuncture could remove an allergy. Furthermore, who would believe that an allergy to fabric, nutrients or other common, everyday, natural and artificial substances could produce such common, everyday dysfunction in the body. I have seen the most amazing things with the NAET technique from instant and permanent removal of daily, intractable headaches to near anaphylactic reaction to fish. I am delighted to have participated in the seminar. There is more than "something to it".

Robert J. Rowen, M.D.
Anchorage, Alaska.

I have treated patients from age two months to 70 years old and find enormous pleasure in watching how their lives change from such simple acupuncture techniques. One says, "I felt as if I was let out of jail!" Another describes it as, "escape from allergy hell." My patients' improvement in health, mood and behavior are, in some cases, incredibly profound and the credit goes to the Nambudripad's Allergy Elimination Technique. Thank you Devi, for a technique that so quickly transforms so many lives.

Carolyn Reuben, L.Ac.
Sacramento, California

Dr. Devi Nambudripad's Allergy Elimination Technique combined with acupuncture, kinesiology, and chiropractic techniques is truly a revolutionary concept in the area of nutrition, allergy and energy work. Concepts of reprogramming nutritional and emotional systems will open a new whole area of how the mind and body function. This absolutely changes negative reaction, not only to food and environmental substances, but to the dental materials also. This knowledge of reprogramming the brain's negative pattern has changed my practice for ever. I am deeply grateful to Devi for sharing this knowledge with me, and I have no doubt that very soon this will change medical and nutritional history.

Vaughn T. Harada, DDS-Dental Acupuncture
Malibu Canyon, California

By using N.A.E.T. treatment I have been able to help our patients eliminate allergies that have been with them since childhood. Thank you Dr. Devi for sharing this miraculous technique!

Sandi Ihlen, R.N.
Anchorage, Alaska

Three years ago I began using Dr. Devi's Allergy Elimination Technique. Ever since that time I have had great success in eliminating allergies to all food, mold, yeast, fungus and dust. I really can't imagine practicing without it now. I look forward to treating those difficult and sometimes baffling cases of chronic fatigue and depression with flu like symptoms, "brainfog," hyperactivity, migraines, PMS, etc. I have learned that many of these patients with their puzzling conditions wear out welcome at doctors' offices because of the difficulty in treating them effectively and safely. These are often the patients with hidden food allergies and environmental hypersensitivities. It is gratifying to be able to clear their debilitating health problems and restore hope after decades of despair.

Dr. Arthur I Cushing, D.C.
Gardiner, Maine

Dr. Devi's techniques represent a profound understanding of the body's reset mechanism which allows the allergic patient to return to normal function. This is an easily tolerated, systematic approach which shows excellent results in clinical practice.

Dr. Randol J. Christman, L.Ac.
Kihei, Maui

My patients ages 6 weeks to 65 are astonished at their results from the Nambudripad's Allergy Elimination Treatment with acupuncture. Their chronic problems have "magically" disappeared.

Lesley Migdali, L.Ac.
Inglewood, California

My wife's irritating, impossible Christmas tree allergy was eliminated by Dr. Devi Nambudripad's fantastic acupuncture discoveries. Her method will revolutionize the current medical approach to allergy treatment for all people.

Dr. Stanley Y. Inouye, D.D.S., M.S.D.
Sacramento, California

Acupuncture using Nambudripad's Allergy Elimination Techniques gives me great satisfaction in treating my patients. My patients and I love the results with NAET....it brings acupuncture into the 21st century.

Denis Alvino, OMD., L.Ac.
Los Angeles, California

BIBLIOGRAPHY

Abehsera, Michel, ed. Healing Ourselves. New York, 1973.

Austin, Mary. Acupuncture Therapy. New York, 1972.

Allergy Foundation of America, 801 Second Ave, New York, NY, 10017

American Medical Association Committee on Rating of Mental and Physical Impairments. Guides to the Evaluation of Permanent Impairment. N.P., 1971

Beeson, Paul B., M.D. and McDermott, Walsh, M.D., eds. Textbook of Medicine. 12th edition, Philadelphia, 1967.

Brodal, A., M.D. Neurological Anatomy in Relation to Clinical Medicine. 2nd ed. New York.

Cerrat, Paul L., "Does Diet Affect the Immune System?" RN, Vol. 53, pp. 67-70 (June 1990).

Collins, Douglas, R. M.D. Illustrated Diagnosis of Systematic Diseases. Philadelphia, 1972.

Daniels, Lucille, M.A. and Catherine Wothingham, Ph.D. Muscle Testing Techniques Of manual Examination.3rd ed. Philadelphia, 1972

Eastland Press, Chicago. Acupuncture, A Comprehensive Test, 1981

Elliot, Frank, A., F.R.C.P. Clinical Laboratory. Philadelphia, 1959

Fazir, Claude A., M.D. parents Guide to Allergy in Children. Doubleday & Co. Inc. Garden City, N.Y. 1973

Foreign Language Press, Beijing. Essentials Of Chinese Acupuncture, Beijing.

Fuelton, Shaton. The Allergy Self Help Book. Rodale Books, Pennsylvania, 1983

Fujihara, Ken, and Hays, Nancy. Common Health Complaints. Oriental Healing Arts Institute, 1982.

Golos, Natalie, and Frances. Coping With Your Allergies, Simon and Schuster, New York.

Goodheart, George, J. Applied Kinesiology, N.P., 1964

Goodheart, George, J. Applied Kinesiology, 1970 Research Manual, 8th ed. N.P., 1971

Goodheart, George, J. Applied Kinesiology, Workshop Manual. N.P. 1972

Goodheart, George, J. Applied Kinesiology,1973 Research Manual. 9th ed. N.P., 1973

Goodheart, George, J. Applied Kinesiology,1974 Research Manual. N.P., 1974

Graziano, Joseph. Footsteps to Better Health, N.P., 1973

Gray, Henry, F.R.S. Anatomy of the Human Body. 27th, 34th, and 38th ed. Philadelphia, 1961

Guyton, Arthur, C. Textbook of Medical Physiology, 2nd ed. Philadelphia, 1961

Hepler, Opal, E., Ph.D., M.D. Manual of Clinical Laboratory Methods. 4th ed. Illinois, 1962.

Hsu, Hong-Yen, Ph.D. Chinese Herb Medicine and Therapy.

Hsu, Hong-Yen, Ph.D. Commonly Used Chinese Herb Formulas with Illustrations. Oriental Healing Arts Institute, 1982.

Hsu, Hong-Yen, Ph.D. Natural Healing With Chinese Herbs. Oriental Healing Arts Institute, 1982.

Heuns, Him-Che. Handbook of Chinese Herbs and Formulae. Vol V. Los Angeles, 1985.

Kirschmann J.D. with Dunne, L.J. Nutrition Almanac 2nd ed. McGraw Hill Book Co. Copyright 1984.

Lawson-Wood, Denis, F.A.C.A. and Lawson-Wood, Joyce. The Five Elements of Acupuncture and Chinese Massage. 2nd ed. Northamptonshire, 1973.

Lyght, Charles, E., M.D. and John M. Trapnell, M.D., eds. The Merck Manual. 11th ed. Rahway, N.J., 1966.

MacKarness, Richard. The Hazards of Hidden Allergies.

Mindell Earl. Vitamin Bible. Warner Books Copyright 1985.

Moss, Louis, M.D. Acupuncture and You. New York, 1964.

Palos, Stephan. The Chinese Art of Healing. New York, 1972.

Peking Medicine health Publishing Co., 1980. The Treatment of 100 Common Diseases.

Pennington & Church. Food Values of Portions Commonly Used. J.B. Lippincott Company. Copyright 1985

Randolph, Theron, G.M.D. An Alternative Approach to Allergies. Lippincott and Conwell, N.Y. 1980

Rapp, Doris. Allergy and your Family. Sterling Publishing Co., Inc. New York, 1980

Shanghai College of Traditional Chinese Medicine. Acupuncture, a Comprehensive Text.

Sierra, Ralph, U. Chiropractic Handbook of Applied Neurology. Mexico, 1956.

Smith, John, H., D.C. Applied Kinesiology and the Specific Muscle Balancing Technique.

Somekh, Emile, M.D. The Complete Guide To Children's Allergies. Pinnacle Books, Inc. 1979.

Stoner, Fred, D.C. The Eclectic Approach to Chiropractic.

Thie, John, F., D.C. with Mary Marks. Touch for Health.

Zong, Linda. "Chinese Internal Medicine," lecture at SAMRA University, Los Angeles, CA. 1985

Case Histories from the Author's private practice.

INDEX

Acne 137, 140, 141, 201, 223, 250, 315, 316, 317, 319

Alcoholism 19, 280, 330

Alzheimer's Disease 18

Amnesia 18

Anemia 236, 320, 324, 325, 329, 330

Angina 206, 226, 229, 230, 232, 285

Anorexia 142, 204, 293

Arteriosclerosis 226, 228, 330, 336

Arthritis 16, 24, 30, 32, 33, 35, 46, 47, 83, 100, 114, 134, 137, 155, 168, 200, 214, 222, 225, 234, 235, 236, 237, 238, 241, 243, 268, 269, 286, 327, 331

Asthma 2, 3, 7, 8, 15, 16, 21, 22, 28, 29, 30, 31, 34, 37, 42, 43, 45, 47, 50, 51, 53, 56, 63, 83, 86, 87, 98, 102, 113,114, 122, 132, 133, 137, 158, 185, 192, 193, 194, 195, 196, 197, 199, 200, 202, 203, 204, 206, 212, 223, 235, 239, 240, 243, 246, 247, 250, 258, 263, 264, 265, 270, 279, 286, 303, 306, 327, 332, 338, 339

Athlete's Foot 35, 48, 49

Backache 16, 20, 37, 179, 203, 215, 216, 237, 281, 282, 306, 326, 327, 328, 329

Bad Breath 137, 142, 208

Belching 114, 137, 196, 209, 211, 218

Bell's Palsy 199

Bladder Infection 2, 34, 105, 215

Blindness 251, 315